Fill in

MW00979664

A Practical Guide to Healthy Teeth

D R. V I C T O R S T E R L I N G

Addison-Wesley Publishers

Don Mills, Ontario • Reading, Massachusetts • Menlo Park, California • New York
Wokingham, England • Amsterdam • Bonn • Sydney
• Singapore • Tokyo
Madrid • San Juan

Editor: Loral Dean

Copy Editor: Susan Berg

Production Editor: Suzanne Payne

Design and Art Direction: Mary Opper

Cover Design: Mary Opper

Cover Illustration: Doug Martin

Inside Illustration: Gary Clement

Canadian Cataloguing in Publication Data
Sterling, Victor, 1956–
Fill in the gaps : a practical guide to healthy teeth

Includes index.
ISBN 0–201–57584–1

1. Teeth – Care and hygiene. 2. Dentistry – Popular works.
I. Title.

RK61.S86 1991   617.6 C91–093893–8

This book contains recycled product and is acid free.
Printed and bound in Canada.

A B C D E F – ALG – 96 95 94 93 92 91

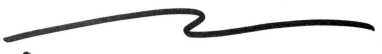

Contents

To Carolyn, David and Cara with gratitude and love.

ACKNOWLEDGMENTS

Many thanks to Loral Dean, my editor, for accommodating my busy practice schedule and working many weekends on the edits.

Many thanks to Jackie Gross, of Addison-Wesley for believing in this project. Also many thanks to all of the people at Addison-Wesley who contributed to the production of this book.

Thanks to my colleagues Drs. James M. Kerr, Murray Chantler, Gordon Nikiforuk, Stanley Markin, David Eller and my partner Steven Nadel for their comments and suggestions.

Many thanks to my wife Carolyn for tirelessly deciphering my scribbles and making them word processible.

Thanks to Risa Shiff for typing parts of the manuscript.

And of course many thanks to David and Cara, for being patient and behaving while Daddy was working on THE BOOK.

Finally thanks to all my patients past, present and future for allowing me to help them and making my job a pleasure.

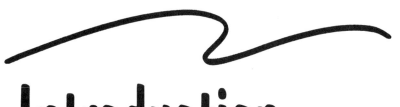

Introduction

Why a book on dentistry?

A well-groomed businessman is sitting in my dental chair. I have just outlined the treatment he requires and explained its pros and cons. I ask if he has any questions. "No," he replies, "everything is quite clear." I leave the room. Immediately he turns to my assistant and asks, "What is he going to do to me?"

Why does it always happen this way? It's certainly not because this man is not intelligent. He has just come from a meeting where he presented a five-year plan for a multinational company. I think that he didn't hear a word I said because of his own anxiety and apprehension. There's something about a dental chair that causes intelligent men and women to suspend their normal thought processes. A dental office is not a good place to learn about dentistry. Hence this book. In my years as a practising dentist, I have noticed over and over again how poorly informed the general public is about dentistry. Most dentists have rows of pamphlets and leaflets in their offices to which they encourage their patients to help themselves. But how many actually do? In my experience, not many. The pamphlets and brochures in my office sit there week after week, year after year, collecting dust.

It's not that people aren't interested in the health of their teeth and what happens while they are sitting in a dentist's chair. A long list of dental assistants and dentists' receptionists will back me up on that statement! But it's become clear to me over the years that the blizzard of dental pamphlets I provide is not the answer. And what I tell my patients in my office frequently goes in one ear and out the other. What people need is a clearly written sourcebook they can consult in the calm and comfort of their own homes.

I searched for a book to recommend to my patients. I found the bookstores full of books on every imaginable subject — every subject that is, except dentistry.

So I wrote this book to explain in plain language for the consumer, what a dentist can and cannot do for you. It is intended to provide you with a lifetime guide to keeping your teeth healthy.

Who should read this book?

Anyone who has a mouth. Notice I said a mouth, not teeth. More than a third of adults over the age of sixty-five have no natural teeth remaining. This is a shame — and completely preventable — as this book will explain. But even if you have no natural teeth at all, this book can help you. It will illustrate different methods of tooth replacement and a range of solutions to problems faced by people with no teeth of their own.

For the rest of you who do have all or most of your own teeth, this book will help you keep them healthy, even if you live to be one hundred. The key to healthy teeth is prevention, not treatment. A healthy mouth doesn't happen by accident. It's the happy result of consistent, regular home care and professional care over many years. It's the payoff for a lifetime of good communication and cooperation between you and your dentist.

How should you read this book?

This book is written in a logical sequence. In Chapter 1, I focus on the personal care of your teeth, and how you can maintain your teeth and prevent tooth decay through meticulous home care. In Chapter 2, I talk about your relationship with your dentist, beginning with how to choose a dentist and what you can expect from him or her. In the next chapter, **Your Dentist and the Tools of the Trade**, I discuss the technology your dentist uses. This chapter addresses the important subject of pain in the dentist's chair. In the final chapter, I discuss the many branches of dentistry. From basic restorative dentistry (filling cavities) to orthodontics (moving and straightening teeth), periodontics (the treatment of gum disease), prosthodontics (replacing teeth), root canals, implants, dentures, specialized dentistry for children and the elderly — it's all there.

I don't expect anyone to read this book from start to finish as though it were a novel. It is intended as an easy-to-use sourcebook to answer your questions and concerns about your teeth. It's organized to help you find the information you need quickly and simply. You can use the Contents page at the beginning of the book, the Glossary and Index at the back of the book, or the subheads and cross-references within the body of the book to guide you to the information you require. The many illustrations and cartoons throughout the book are there to clarify what I'm discussing and to add a light touch. Each chapter and section contains enough information on its own to answer most questions. This means there is some overlap and repetition from section to section, but it's the only way to make this a quick resource book. Besides, isn't repetition the father of learning?

Don't use this book to diagnose your dental problems!
I want to stress an important point. This book is not intended to be used as a self-diagnosis manual. **Please do not make decisions concerning your condition based on this book alone.** Only your dentist, backed by years of experience and formal education, is qualified to diagnose oral disorders. This book is intended only to give you enough information to know what to ask your dentist, to help you understand the answers, and to clarify some of the suggestions you get.

I have used plain, easy-to-understand terminology wherever possible. However, dentistry is a highly specialized field and from time to time I have had to use words that are less familiar. I have tried to explain foreign or unusual words wherever I use them. If you do come across something that you don't understand, look it up in the Glossary at the end of the book.

Now, without further ado, read for your health!

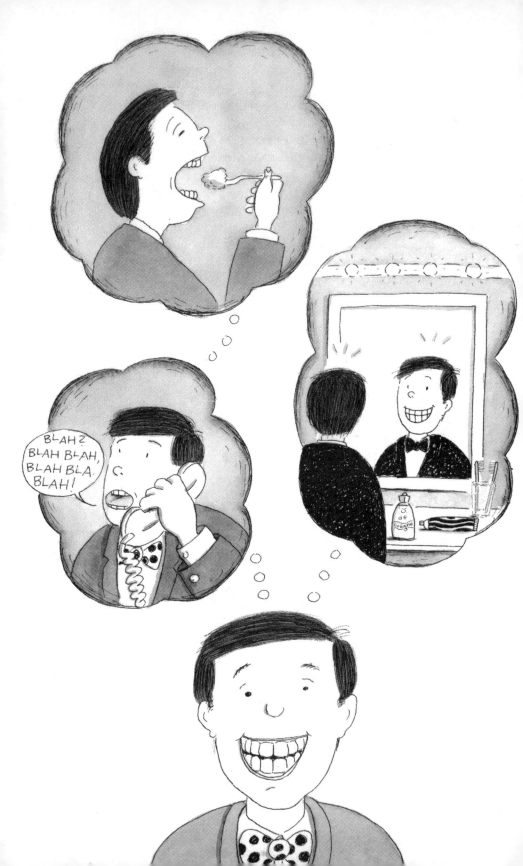

You and your Teeth

Your teeth and you

Think about your mouth for a moment. You use it every day for speaking, for chewing your food, for conveying messages with your smiles or frowns. You laugh with it, you cry with it, you make first and lasting impressions with it. Yet most people don't think about the welfare of their mouth and teeth until something goes wrong. Not until a toothache awakens them at night or they feel an unpleasant sensation while munching on their favorite snack do they finally quit procrastinating and make an appointment with a dentist. Then and only then do they put themselves in the hands of the dentist and say, fix it. And when the visit is over and the urgency taken care of, they forget about their mouth and teeth until the next emergency comes up.

Yet healthy teeth are crucial to your appearance and to the overall health and well-being of your body. Missing, broken, or decayed teeth can change an otherwise attractive person into an unkempt, sad-looking wreck of a human being. If neglected, an infected tooth can spread its poison throughout the body. Loose or missing teeth reduce your chewing efficiency and make you gulp your food in chunks. This can lead to digestive problems. If a sufficient number of teeth are missing or out of their proper place, pain and discomfort can arise in the muscles of the face and in jaw joints.

Whether or not they ever enter your thoughts, your mouth and teeth are very important. Taking good care of your teeth doesn't have to take a lot of time or effort. What it does take are good, daily habits.

Why is it important to keep my teeth?

Good reason #1: maintaining proper digestion

The long process of digestion begins in your mouth when you think of food and begin salivating. It ends when the food waste products are eliminated from your body.

The saliva in your mouth contains enzymes. Enzymes are chemicals that break down food into its building blocks. Your body gets its energy and nutrients from these building blocks. The enzymes can work efficiently only if the food is broken down into tiny pieces. If your teeth don't do a proper job of chewing and breaking down your food, big chunks of food will travel down to your stomach. This means that your stomach and intestines have to work harder, and that less energy and fewer nutrients are extracted from the food you eat.

Good reason #2: preventing pain and infection

Neglected teeth decay and frequently become infected. An infected tooth leads to an abscess, which is an accumulation of pus at the tip of the root. An abscessed tooth, like any infection in the body, causes pain and sometimes fever. An infection in one tooth can spread to neighboring teeth. And untreated infections in the mouth can spread to other parts of the body such as the sinuses and the chest cavity. Periodontal (gum) disease is a chronic infection that causes heavy stress on the body's immune system. Untreated, it can seriously complicate some heart conditions.

Good reason #3: maintaining healthy jaw joints and facial muscles

When teeth are missing or misaligned, the upper and lower jaws don't mesh properly. This puts a strain on the jaw joints located just in front of each ear. In time, these joints develop cracking noises and can become very painful. The face muscles that control the movement of the jaws during speech and chewing have to work extra hard under these conditions. Eventually this leads to painful spasms in these muscles. Collectively, these conditions are called TMJ Dysfunction Syndrome. TMJ Syndrome is a debilitating condition that can cause severe, sometimes unbearable pain around the jaw joints and lower part of the face. Often the condition takes the form of recurring migraine headaches.

Good reason #4: looking good

Let's forget about medical sense for a moment and talk about something we can all relate to — good looks. Healthy teeth help people look their best. A full set of well-shaped, straight teeth is as basic to good looks as good posture and proper weight. I'll go further: Attractive teeth are probably the single most important factor affecting appearance. *Nothing* undermines a person's looks more than unsightly or missing teeth. A healthy set of teeth fills out a person's cheeks and lips. Properly aligned teeth maintain the correct vertical height of the face. Sparkling teeth and pink gums are essential to a vibrant smile. And, like it or not, the world we live in places enormous emphasis on appearance. Fortunately, people don't have to be Hollywood handsome to have lovely smiles. All they need are healthy teeth and gums.

Good reason #5: bolstering self-esteem

A confident smile radiating from a healthy body is a great psychological boost. It's the best antidote I know to a bad day. It can bolster your self-esteem immeasurably. Taking a few minutes every day to look after your teeth can boost your psyche by allowing you some time for yourself. Our lives are busy with family responsibilities and job pressures, and it feels good to take time on a regular basis to do something purely self-centred. Enjoy the few minutes a day you devote to the welfare of your gums and teeth. Don't think of it as a chore — think of it as pampering yourself.

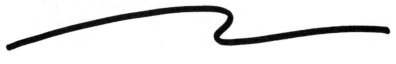

Your diet and your teeth

We are what we eat, and what we eat is crucial to the health of our teeth and mouth. According to Canada's Food Guide, we need foods every day from all four major food groups. The four groups are fruits and vegetables; breads and cereals; milk and milk products; meat, fish, poultry, and alternates (dried peas, beans, lentils, nuts, and seeds). Choosing foods from each of these groups every day provides people with the benefit of the more than fifty nutrients essential for growth and good health.

Of these fifty or more nutrients, the following are the most important to the health of the mouth and teeth.

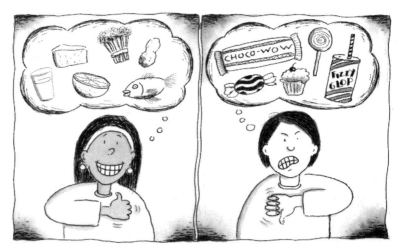

● **Protein**
Protein builds and repairs soft tissues such as gums and builds antibodies, the blood components that fight infection.

One of the least expensive sources of high-quality protein is milk. One cup of milk has the same amount of protein as one egg or one ounce (thirty grams) of meat. Meat, fish, poultry, and eggs are all high in protein content. Beans, peas, and lentils provide additional alternatives.

● **Calcium, phosphorus, and magnesium**
These minerals help form and maintain strong bones and teeth.

Calcium is found in milk and milk products such as cheeses, yogurt, and ice cream.

Magnesium is found in red meats, peanut butter, nuts, and whole grains.

Phosphorus is found in poultry, fish, and meats.

● **Vitamin C**
Vitamin C maintains healthy teeth and gums.

It is found in citrus fruits and their juices, and in fruits and vegetables such as broccoli, Brussels sprouts, green and red peppers, strawberries, cauliflower, sweet potatoes, and tomatoes.

● **Vitamin A**
Vitamin A aids normal bone and tooth development, and healthy skin.

It is found in organ meats such as liver; milk; carrots; dark green vegetables such as spinach and broccoli; and fruits such as peaches, cantaloupe, tomatoes, and watermelon.

● **Vitamin D**
Vitamin D helps the body utilize calcium and phosphorus, which are essential to the formation and maintenance of healthy bones and teeth.

Vitamin D is added to all liquid milk sold in Canada. Milk

products such as yogurt, cheese, and ice cream are not fortified with vitamin D. So to meet the requirements for this vitamin, you must drink liquid milk (or take supplementary vitamin D tablets).

A balanced diet builds a strong body that is able to defend itself against infections and bacterial invasions and maintain a strong immune system. Good nutrition helps the body to repair itself more easily, too. Minor irritations heal faster in the presence of a good supply of proteins and vitamins.

Will eating sweets ruin my teeth?

Children often ask me wistfully if they can eat all the sweets they want if they brush right afterward. Well, I wish I could say yes, but I cannot. The answer — sorry, kids — is a resounding *no*.
Why?

Reason #1:
The time it takes to eat or drink a sweet snack is heaven for the millions of decay-producing bacteria inside your mouth. Brushing, even immediately, won't get you off the hook. Your mouth is crammed with hard-to-get-at nooks and crannies. You rarely reach all of them in a single brushing.

Reason #2:
Candy, packaged snack foods, pastries, desserts, soft drinks, and all those other sugar-filled treats are nutritionally empty foods. The more you eat and drink of them, the more empty calories you consume. Sugar doesn't build strong bones and muscles. It does nothing for you except perhaps give you a quick (and fleeting) hit of energy.

The best (and worst) time for a sugar hit

As a general rule, keep away from sweets as much as possible. When you do indulge, do so at the end of a meal. When you're finishing a meal, your mouth is busily producing a lot of saliva. Saliva is nature's way of keeping your teeth clean: It helps wash the sugar off your teeth. Then, when you've finished your sweets, brush your teeth as soon as you can.

The worst time to indulge your sweet tooth is in the evening before you go to bed — even if you brush afterward. Why? Because it's almost impossible to get at every area in your mouth in a single brushing. And, your mouth produces very little saliva as you sleep — unless you dream about food every night! This means that the sugar remnants are not washed off and just sit there, feeding the decay-producing bacteria throughout the long night hours.

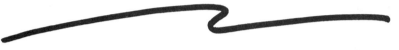

You and the care of your teeth

Brushing

How often should I brush my teeth?

You should brush your teeth at least twice a day. Perhaps that sounds reasonable to you. But you'd be surprised how many people come into my office telling me they brush their teeth once a week — or even less often. I have one patient who calmly announced on his first visit that he brushed his teeth twice a year. (It wouldn't have surprised me if he'd added, "whether my teeth need it or not.") One look inside his mouth convinced me he wasn't kidding. And if I hadn't had a cold at the time, I wouldn't even have had to check out his mouth. My receptionist, whose nasal passages were functioning normally that day, picked up the patient's scent before he said a word — while he was still outside in the waiting room!

This person has been a patient of mine now for seven years and, thanks to my salutary influence, he now brushes every other day. I guess I can't complain: that's ninety times more often per year than before he came to my office!

Seriously, there is a scientific basis for my advice to brush at least twice a day. Studies show that plaque takes twenty-four hours to form. So why not brush once every twenty-four hours, you may ask. You could — it's certainly better than every two days or twice a year — but this assumes you brush perfectly every time. Nobody is that good (and that includes me). You need to give yourself a second chance. The second time you brush, chances are you'll cover spots you missed the first time round. Of course, a third and fourth time would improve your chances even more. The more frequent the brushing, the faster the sugar is cleared from the mouth, giving decay-causing bacteria that much less time to feast. But you have to be practical, too. I'm not trying to turn you into a Mad Tooth Brusher, excusing yourself from boardrooms and conference calls to rush to a sink to attend to your teeth!

Brush after breakfast and before going to bed.

Brushing in the morning right after breakfast is important because it gets rid of nighttime plaque buildup as well as breakfast food in your mouth. And it will give you a fresh, clean mouth until lunchtime.

The last thing you should do at night before going to bed is brush your teeth. Why is it so important to make tooth-

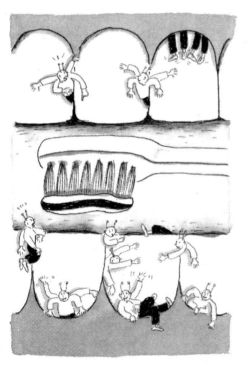

brushing your last activity of the day? Because when you are sleeping, the bacteria inside your mouth are wide awake. Bacteria are tiny, microscopic-sized, living organisms that exist almost everywhere. They live inside your mouth and your intestines and all over your skin. It may come as a shock to you, but having some bacteria cohabiting with you like this is quite normal. But if you don't clean your teeth before you go to sleep, you're inviting all those bacteria living in your mouth to an all-night party, feasting on all the leftover bits and pieces of food in your mouth. They don't need a formal invitation! While you're peacefully sleeping, the bugs are having a ball eating, reproducing, and leaving behind waste products that, over time, dissolve your teeth and destroy your gums. No wonder your mouth feels like the bottom of a birdcage in the morning! Don't give the bugs the opportunity. Never go to sleep without first cleaning your teeth.

Choosing a toothbrush

Medium to soft is best.

The toothbrush you use is very important. Always select a medium or a soft brush (unless your dentist instructs you to do otherwise for some specific reason). Most people choose a brush that is too hard, thinking that the harder they brush, the better they will be scrubbing their teeth.

They're wrong.

Over my years of peering inside people's mouths, I've seen a lot of damage done by toothbrushes that are too hard. I've seen severely receded gums and deep grooves cut into the sides of patients' teeth. It's hard to believe that a brush can cut a groove in something as hard as a tooth but, believe me, it can and does. These grooves and notches make teeth very sensitive and fragile. Some of my older patients have cut such deep and wide wedge-shaped grooves that yelling "Timber!" is about all that's needed to make their entire set of teeth fall down. Until recently, this kind of damage was very difficult to treat. Now it can be treated with some of the newer bonding materials. But you can save yourself a lot of grief and your dentist a lot of work by using a medium or soft brush.

A long handle and a small head works well.

The size of your toothbrush is important, too. Choose a brush with a long handle and a small head (the head is the part where the bristles are). You might think that the bigger and bushier the brush, the better it will clean. Not so. Teeth are irregular in shape, and they follow the curve of your jaw. A large brush can clean only the high spots of your teeth. A small brush will get into all the valleys between your teeth. And it will force you to spend more time brushing — all to the good! The bristles of the brush should be rounded. Most brushes today have rounded-off individual bristles, and that will be indicated on the package.

Choosing a toothpaste

Toothpastes are a very personal matter. The extensive marketing done by toothpaste manufacturers has created a lot of brand loyalty.

When you choose a toothpaste, stick with the three or four leading brands. All of these toothpastes have low abrasion levels, which means that they will not remove tooth material from your teeth during brushing. These toothpastes also contain fluoride, which is an important aid in making your teeth more cavity-resistant. Be sure that any toothpaste you use carries the American or Canadian Dental Association's seal of approval. This is your guarantee that the paste has met these associations' standards.

Some newer toothpastes advertise themselves as calculus (tartar) fighters. These toothpastes contain pyrophosphate ions, which prevent the formation of large calculus crystals. They're fine —as far as they go. They *do* reduce new calculus as it is forming. But any calculus deposits already there are unaffected and must be removed by your hygienist or dentist. It is important to remember that toothpastes only *help* to reduce calculus and are no substitute for regular cleaning visits.

From time to time, toothpastes show up on the market promising whiter teeth, removal of stains, and a flurry of other wonders. Be careful with these. Some of them are very abrasive. Some are poorly tested and may discolor any white fillings you may have inside your mouth. If you are tempted to try any of these new brands, check with your dentist first. Your teeth will thank you, I promise you.

Junior toothpastes

Junior toothpastes are special formulations intended to appeal to youngsters. They provide more gentle cleaning action with minimal abrasion. They contain less detergent, reducing accidental gagging caused by foam. They come in mild flavors for the younger palate and they contain extra fluoride for growing teeth. They also come in zippy packaging designed to make kids want to brush more often. I'm all for these toothpastes because they do seem to promote more frequent brushing — at my house and among my younger patients, anyway.

How to brush

Small is beautiful.

Brush in small sections, one or two teeth at a time (one more reason to use a small-headed brush).

Position your toothbrush at a forty-five-degree angle to the tooth. Place the bristles inside the cuff of gum around the tooth, without forcing — just feel them go in. Gently jiggle the brush from side to side while rolling it upward toward the edge of the tooth. The idea is to get the plaque out of the cuff and into your mouth where you can rinse it out.

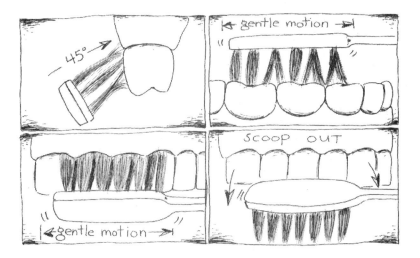

To repeat: Place the brush into the cuff of the gum and very gently vibrate from side to side; then roll up and out. **Important:** Do not jiggle from side to side too vigorously. Be gentle. You just want to scoop out soft plaque from the inside of the groove or cuff of the gum. Remember my "Timber!" story and think "massage," not "scrub." You don't want your teeth falling down like trees a few years from now!

Repeat this gentle action on the top, on the bottom, on the face-side, and on the tongue-side of every tooth. Try to change your mental image of brushing your teeth: Instead of picturing your brush cleaning your entire set of teeth, picture it cleaning each tooth individually. Brushing like this takes a little more time but once you get the hang of it and it becomes a habit — a good habit — you'll do it automatically.

The reason you need to brush your teeth every day is to remove the soft plaque and debris from your teeth — before it hardens into calculus (tartar). Soft plaque undisturbed by brushing will harden into tartar in about twenty-four hours. Once this happens, a toothbrush is useless. You'll never remove tartar with a brush — only a dentist or hygienist has the tools for that.

Flossing

What is floss?
Floss is strong thread that you slide between your teeth and use to scoop soft plaque gently off the side of each tooth.

If I carefully brush my teeth in small sections, tooth by tooth, at least twice a day, do I have to floss too?
Yes. Flossing is essential. Brushing alone only cleans the cheek- and tongue-sides of your teeth. To clean in-between your teeth, you have to floss.

Think about it this way. Each tooth has five surfaces: top, cheek, tongue, and the two surfaces touching the neighboring teeth. If you don't floss, you are cleaning only three of these five surfaces — only sixty percent of them. The other forty percent of your teeth get cleaned occasionally or not at all. I think these numbers speak for themselves, don't you?

Choosing a floss
You have two basic choices: waxed and unwaxed.

Waxed floss

● Its pluses: Waxed floss slips more easily between the teeth than unwaxed floss and doesn't shred as readily.

● Its minuses: Some wax may rub off the floss and cake on the teeth, creating an ideal spot for bacteria to attach themselves and flourish.

Unwaxed floss

● Its pluses: It is more absorbent than waxed floss and it leaves no waxy residue.

● Its minuses: Some people find unwaxed floss harder to place between their teeth. It also tends to shred more easily.

Flavored floss is available now as are some new easy-glide fibre products. Feel free to try any of these products. Whatever works for you — and gets you to clean that neglected forty percent of your teeth — is great by me!

How to floss

Break off eight to ten inches (twenty to twenty-five centimetres) of floss. Wrap the ends around the middle finger of each hand, leaving two to three inches (eight to ten centimetres) of floss between your fingers. Then, using your thumbs and index fingers for your top teeth, or both of your index fingers for your bottom teeth, guide the floss in-between each tooth. Go in-between each two teeth twice,

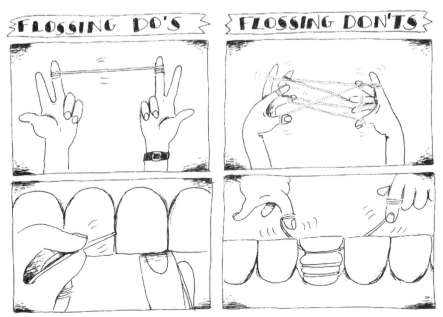

once to clean the side of one tooth of the pair, the second time to clean the side of the other tooth.

Move the floss past the contact point between the teeth (the tight point where teeth touch each other) and down into the groove of the gum. Then press the floss against one tooth while drawing it upward. The object is to scoop the plaque gently off the side of the tooth. Go back into the same spot, but this time press the floss against the other of the two teeth. Draw it upward, cleaning the side of that tooth. You may have to jiggle the floss a bit to get it past the contact points but once it's past, don't keep sawing away at your gums. Soft plaque is ... soft. There's no need for overkill. Once again: **Be gentle.**

How often should I floss?
Ideally twice a day, each time you brush. But for practical purposes, once a day before bed will do.

What if I can't get my fingers in-between all my teeth?
You are not alone with this problem. Many people, because of age, infirmity, or lack of agility can't floss exactly as I have described. If you have a problem, you might try a floss handle or wand, which is Y-shaped. The forked end goes into your mouth and the two arms of the fork take the place of your fingers. You tie your floss from one arm of the wand to the other and use one hand to reach back to those hard-to-get-at areas.

Rubber tips, water irrigators, and other toothcare paraphernalia

Many toothbrushes have a funny-looking rubber tip on one end. What's it for?
It's for massaging your gums.

Why should I massage my gums?
Massaging stimulates circulation in your gums, which may speed up the removal of toxic substances from the mas-

saged areas as well as bring new antibodies and infection-fighting immune cells into the area. This is great news for your gums. It allows them to fight periodontal disease more effectively and speed up the healing of your gums after any periodontal damage.

How do I use the rubber tip?

Lay the rubber tip between your teeth, on your gums. Place the pointy tip in the direction of the chewing surfaces of your teeth, not into the gum. Exert gentle pressure — just enough to make the gum under the rubber tip become pale. Release the pressure. Blood now rushes back into the area, the paleness disappears, and the gum becomes pink again. Repeat all around your mouth. You should massage your gums in this fashion once a day after you floss. If this seems too much trouble, talk to your dentist about your gums. You may be one of those people whose flossing and cleaning efforts result in terrific, healthy gums and you may not need the additional massages. But they definitely can't hurt.

Should I use an electric water irrigator?

Electric water irrigators spray pulsating jets of water or other liquid through a small nozzle attached to a handle. They're great for cleaning around orthodontic braces, crowns, and bridgework. They're also good for dislodging stubborn bits of food and debris stuck in the nooks and crannies of your mouth.

The irrigator's pulsating action is an effective gum massage too, and you can use it to circulate other liquid solutions recommended by your dentist. Some dentists recommend salt-and-water solutions for rinsing your mouth at home after a scaling and cleaning appointment. Others tell their patients to rinse with hydrogen-peroxide solutions to help control gum disease. Water irrigators are ideal for both these purposes.

Water irrigators don't do everything well, however. They don't remove plaque very effectively. For that — sorry — there's no substitute for old-fashioned, manual brushing and flossing.

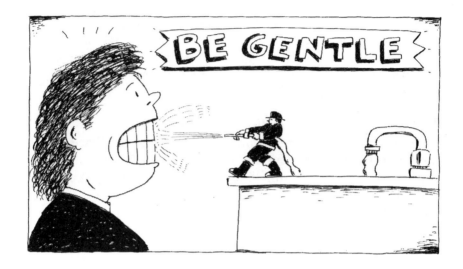

How do I use a water irrigator?

Be gentle. Don't start with the highest control settings the first day you use a water irrigator. You probably won't cause permanent damage, but you may well give yourself sore gums. Ease into it.

Electric toothbrushes

I am not a great fan of electric toothbrushes. My fear is that they promote a lazy attitude toward thorough brushing. People seem to think that letting these brushes buzz around for a few minutes will clean their entire mouth like magic. This is *not* the case. You still have to direct the brush carefully into all areas of your mouth.

However, electric toothbrushes may help handicapped people or people with poor manual dexterity brush more effectively. And recently I have softened my stand against using electric toothbrushes. Why? Because some of my patients have invested between one and two hundred dollars in a rotating-bristle electric toothbrush and are getting great results. Whether the size of their investment has made them more conscientious or whether it's the brush itself, I am not yet sure. The bottom line is this: If the wonders of technology help you get closer to that one hundred percent squeaky-clean state, by all means use them.

What's the best way to clean under a bridge?

Keeping a permanent bridge fastidiously clean is very important. The whole bridge has to be replaced if any of the supporting teeth are lost. Replacing a bridge is expensive at best. At worst, it may be impossible to reconstruct a tooth-supported bridge if a strategic tooth is missing.

But cleaning under a bridge is not always easy. The bridge teeth are joined together and you cannot floss in-between them in the normal fashion. Instead you must get the floss under the bridge between the gum tissue and the underside of the bridge.

Use a floss threader.

A floss threader is a stiff nylon string with a large loop at the end of it. It works like a regular sewing needle threader. Pass the floss through the nylon loop and then slip the nylon string-end under your bridge. Pull it through. Voilà — the floss is under your bridge. Now grasp the two ends of the floss and carefully slide the floss over the sides of the teeth on either side of the bridge, as well as under the bridge itself. A lot of plaque can collect underneath the false teeth of the bridge. The bridge itself won't decay — it's made of metal and porcelain — but the bacteria in plaque may irritate the gum tissues under the bridge.

You can use a "proxy" — an interproximal brush — too.

An interproximal brush is sold as a handle with inter-changeable brush tips. The brush tips are small bristles on a short wire that look something like a pipe cleaner.

Gently place the bristle-end underneath your bridge from the cheek- and tongue-side. Remember, plaque is soft so don't scrape; just gently clean.

Should I use a mouth rinse?

There are a number of plaque-fighting mouth rinses now available commercially. They're useful for reducing plaque — but they're *not* a substitute for brushing and flossing. Plaque sticks to the teeth like putty and *nothing* removes it like thorough brushing and flossing.

Ask your dentist if a plaque rinse is recommended. If so, you can check its effectiveness by using disclosing tablets.

*Use disclosing tablets to find out how well you are
fighting plaque.*
There's an easy way to check how effectively you're getting
rid of plaque. **Disclosing tablets** — available from your
dentist or at a drugstore — are food-dye tablets that selectively stain plaque.

Brush and floss as usual. Then put one disclosing tablet
inside your mouth, chew it thoroughly, and use your tongue
to spread it all around your teeth and gums. Open your
mouth wide and look into a mirror. Most of your tongue,

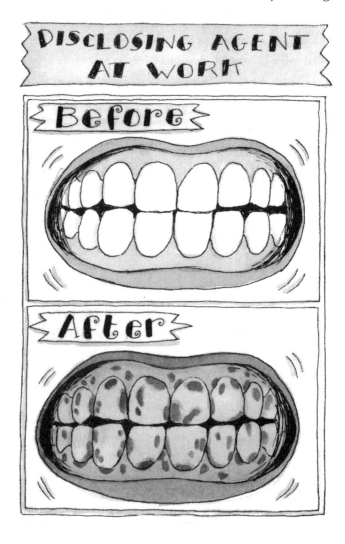

teeth, and gums will be stained a reddish tinge. Look closely at your teeth right around the gumline. Some places will be much more heavily stained than others. These are your problem areas — the spots that are heavily stained are coated with plaque. They are the areas you missed when you brushed and flossed.

Now go back and brush these areas again. And try to remember the problem spots the next time you brush and floss.

Repeat the test every few weeks to see how thoroughly you are cleaning your teeth. But don't do it before an important meeting. The dye takes a few hours to disappear!

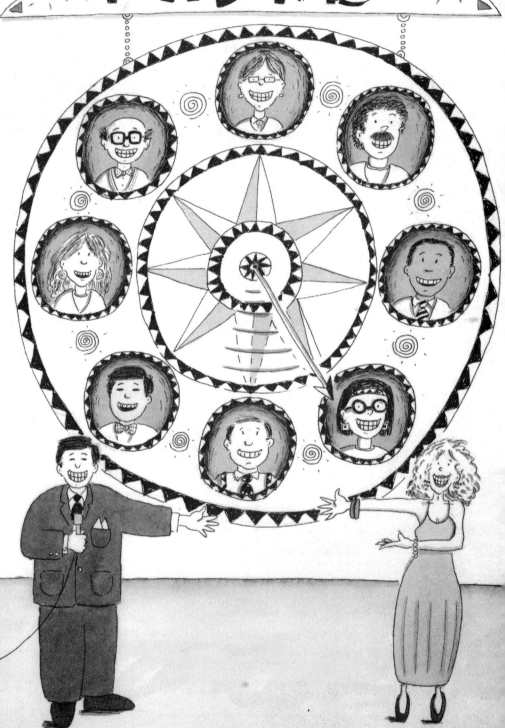

You and
your dentist

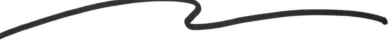

Choosing a dentist

How often should I see a dentist?

Patients often ask me this question. My answer is that there is no specific time interval that fits everyone, because every mouth is different.

Every mouth is different.

I once saw a patient who had not seen a dentist in thirty-seven years. Of course, when I heard this, I foolishly could not resist giving him a sermon. Only after delivering this sermon did I look into his mouth — and found one of the most perfect sets of teeth and gums I have ever seen! Not a filling, a cavity, nor a missing tooth anywhere. His gums were perfect and there was no tartar at all on his teeth. Talk about feeling foolish for speaking too soon!

So what is this patient's best check-up interval — every thirty-seven years? Before we make such a dramatic statement, let's consider what a check-up does. What I look for in your mouth during a check-up are *early* signs of cavities, *early* signs of abscessed teeth, *early* signs of tumors or gum disease, and broken or chipped fillings.

My aim is prevention, not a cure. Because by the time problems get bad enough that you become aware of them through pain or discomfort, their treatment is much more extensive and expensive. The thirty-seven year man is the exception that proves the rule, nothing more. He is highly unusual — and exceptionally lucky.

But he too should start coming for annual checkups — just in case his luck changes.

Only your dentist knows for sure.
Let your dentist decide how often you should see a dentist. As your dentist gets to know you over several visits, he or she will see how quickly you develop cavities, how quickly you form tartar on your teeth, and how rapid and extensive your gum response is to plaque and tartar. All these things are very individual. Every mouth is different, and only after a few visits can your mouth be knowledgeably assessed.

As a general rule I see my patients every six months. However, some patients' oral hygiene, eating habits, and natural body resistance are such that a checkup and light cleaning once a year are enough. Others need to be seen once a month, at least for a while. Gradually this period is extended until I see them every two or three months. If I see continued progress, I cut back on their visits; if I see them backslide, I recommend more frequent visits.

How can I find a good dentist?

Talk to other people.
The best way to find a good dentist is to ask your friends and relatives. Chances are they are seeing someone they like. Remember the saying "birds of a feather stick to-gether"? Your friends are probably a lot like you, and if they like their dentist, chances are you will too.

If you are new in town, look up the local dental association in your phone book. These associations have directories of dentists in different neighborhoods. And they can help you if you have specific needs such as an office with wheelchair access or a dentist who uses general anesthesia.

Should I choose a large, shopping-mall office or a small, single-dentist office?

The new trend in dentistry is large group practices. These are located in busy shopping malls or in storefronts on downtown streets. The advantages to the dentist are shared overhead expenses, greater visibility, and the ability to utilize invested capital over longer hours. The advantages for patients are easier access and more convenient hours. The more traditional type of practice involves a single practitioner in a smaller office, usually not on a main floor, with shorter hours.

So which should you choose?

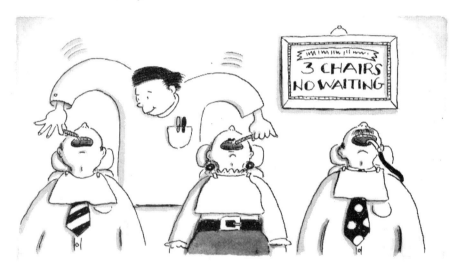

There are advantages to both setups. The storefront location offering convenient, longer hours of service has a rotating team of dentists who work twelve hours a day, six or even seven days a week. You may not see the same dentist for each appointment. And because dentists, like most people, don't particularly like to work late hours or on weekends, there will probably be a rapid turnover in the practice.

The smaller, single-dentist practice may not offer extended hours, but at least every time you go in you will see the same dentist. Only you can decide whether convenience or stability is more important to you.

Sizing up your dentist

Look, feel and listen.

● **Is the office staff friendly and courteous?**
Engage receptionists in small talk. Ask questions about the practice. Chances are greater of poor communication later on, should problems arise, if receptionists are unwilling or too busy to talk to you now.

● **Were you expected? Were you addressed by name?**
You want to be valued as a human being, not treated like just another number that strolled in.

● **Is the waiting room clean and up-to-date?**
A dirty or unkempt reception room may indicate a poor attitude towards cleanliness by the entire staff, including the dentist. You don't want to wonder if the instruments were cleaned and sterilized.

● **Does the dentist see you on time?**
Emergencies and unforeseen circumstances do arise in a dentist's office. But you should be alerted by someone in the office if there is a delay. If the office staff members have no respect for your time, why should they expect you to respect theirs?

● **What kind of questions does the dentist ask you? Is he or she receptive to your questions and concerns?**
A dentist-patient relationship is like any doctor-patient relationship. It depends on trust, mutual respect, and good communication.

Be as critical as you like on your initial visit. It's important for both of you that rapport is established. Be fair, but trust your own judgement. If the vibes are bad, go elsewhere — even if the dentist seems technically competent. There's more to good dentistry than skill with a drill.

After the initial examination appointment, the dentist will draw up a plan of treatment for you. The dentist may simply discuss, at the end of your visit, what needs to be done, if the treatment is simple. If the treatment is more complex, it may entail a second consultation visit to go over the details. During one of these appointments, the dentist should spend some time with you explaining exactly what will be done. It's important to bring up any special concerns that you may have at this time, such as anxiety over treatment, cost, or the amount of time that will be involved. Observe the response to your concerns. Is it empathetic or is it an indication that the dentist just wants to get on to the next appointment?

After one or two initial visits you should have a pretty good idea whether you like and trust this dentist, and whether your personalities mesh. If you feel that the dentist is not suited to your needs, try another. It's perfectly acceptable to ask a dentist's office to forward your records to another one. Usually all that will be transferred, however, are your X-rays.

You will have to pay the first dentist an examination fee, a fee for the X-rays, and possibly a consultation fee if there was a long second consultation appointment. Apart from the X-rays, you will be out-of-pocket perhaps sixty to one hundred and twenty dollars. Over the long term, I think that is a small price to pay to find a dentist who is exactly what you want for you and your loved ones.

Now that you know how to find the perfect dentist, let me mention a few don'ts.

Don't price shop.

I once saw a sign in a dentist's office that read: "Don't look for bargains in parachutes, brain surgery or dentistry." That says it all. Let's face it, qualified dentistry takes skill and time. If a dentist offers a special or a deal, in which of these areas will he compromise? In which would you like him to compromise? Bargains simply don't apply in certain areas of life.

Don't call to find out how much a filling will cost.

When I first started practising dentistry, one of my biggest frustrations was with people calling to see how much a filling would cost. How was I supposed to answer such a

question without knowing anything about the tooth
involved? I would offer a range of fees, but somehow the
caller only heard the lowest number in the range. If I
refused to quote fees over the phone, I would find the
conversation at an end right there. I've figured out how to
deal with this problem now. Whenever my receptionist gets
a call like this, she replies with the question, "How big a
filling do you need?" Almost always, that's all it takes to
make the caller understand that it's impossible to estimate
the fee without seeing exactly what is required in the particular case.

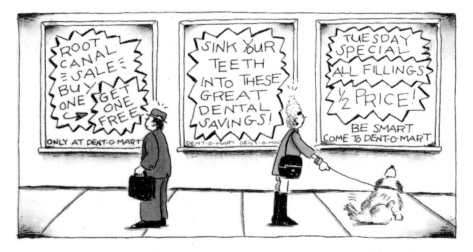

Don't change dentists because of a misunderstanding.

Communication is king in any kind of a relationship,
including the patient-dentist one. If you are not happy with
your present dentist, share your feelings with the dentist
before you make a change. I know this is not always easy,
but often a small misunderstanding compounded by lack of
communication will mushroom into an insurmountable
problem. A ten-minute, honest conversation can often
bring things back on track. Don't be afraid to be direct and
talk about anything, including fees or the attitude of other
people in the office. We dentists are human too. We make
mistakes — and sometimes we are not aware of what goes
on in the reception room. So take a few minutes and talk. If
that doesn't work go ahead and look for another dentist.
Now you'll be doing so with a clear conscience.

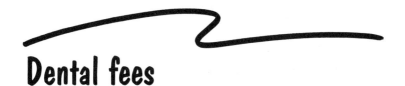

Dental fees

How are dental fees set?

The fees charged by dentists are calculated by considering the amount of time, skill, and risk involved in a given procedure. Most provinces in Canada have dental associations that establish a suggested fee guide for dentists in that province. This fee guide lists hundreds of different procedures and their suggested fees.

This guide is available only to dentists who are members of the association. The guide is updated annually to reflect changes in costs involved in running a dental office. These changes are based on responses that the association receives to a questionnaire it sends to its member dentists.

Not all dentists follow the suggested fee guide.

Dentists are not required to follow this guide. However, most dentists base their fees close to it. Aberrations from the fee guide are usually due to regional economic conditions. For example, there is only one fee guide in the province of Ontario. However, the rent and salaries that a dentist pays in Sarnia are much lower than those paid in downtown Toronto. So dentists in smaller towns generally charge less than dentists in large cities.

Ask what the fees are.

When you are starting with a new dentist, ask whether the fees charged are within the guidelines of the provincial fee guide, or if the dentist charges above it. Remember that the dentist is under no obligation to charge according to the fee guide. The dentist is free to charge what he or she likes — and you are free to take your dental business where you like.

Can I bargain with my dentist?

Usually not. Most dentists' fees are pretty rigid. Every once in a while I get patients who try to get me to reduce my fee because they are having three or four crowns done at once or because they referred their brother-in-law and his family of eight to me. Unfortunately, I must turn them down. Dentistry is not like an assembly line. The laws of mass production do not apply. If a patient needs two crowns, he or she requires twice as much work than if only one crown were done. It's not as if we take two crowns off the shelf and are happy to reduce our inventory. Time, effort, and materials double, so the fee must double too.

Do I have to pay after each appointment?

Although some dentists bill by mail at the end of every month, most offices, including my own, expect payment at the end of each visit. In some cases you may be allowed to pay with a post-dated cheque. Most offices today accept credit cards. If the amount is substantial, you may be able to set up some kind of payment plan. You should arrange such payment plans before your dentist begins the work. Amounts, time period, and interest (if any) should be clearly spelled out in advance to prevent misunderstandings. Most offices will allow short-term payment arrangements. But remember — a dental office is not a bank. The dentist has bills to pay too — and bills that can't be postponed indefinitely.

Dental insurance

Am I charged differently if I have dental insurance?

No. Whether or not you have dental insurance, you pay the same fees. This brings up a point that is often misunderstood by patients. Dental insurance is meant to help offset some or most of your dental expenses. Many patients assume that their dental insurance should cover all of their dental expenses as their provincial health plans cover all of their medical expenses. Unfortunately, it does not work this way. Our government does not pay for universal dental care, and private insurance company coverage is only as good as the premiums your employer pays for the plan. Check your coverage carefully. It may well be only partial. But don't knock it — it's still a lot better than having to pay all your dental fees yourself!

How does dental insurance work?

Dental insurance coverage works like this: Your employer, union, or association goes out and looks for an insurance company that offers the most extensive coverage plan for the least amount of money. Different insurance companies have different plan ranges, and some of the bigger companies offer several levels of coverage.

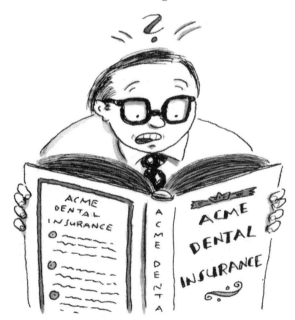

Once your employer or association decides on a plan within its budget, it signs a contract for one year or more to cover all of its employees or members and their dependants.

In general, the more basic the coverage the less expensive it is. As well, coverage that pays for less than the whole dental fee is less expensive than one that covers the full fee. A basic coverage plan has an annual maximum of approximately $750 and pays eighty percent of fees for checkups, basic cleanings, fillings, and extractions. Such a plan does not cover root-canal treatments, crowns, bridges, dentures, orthodontic work, or gum treatments. A top-of-the-line plan pays one hundred percent for all these services with an annual maximum of $10,000. Most plans that I see in my office fall somewhere between these two extremes.

How do insurance companies calculate their reimbursements?

In the contract that your employer signs with an insurance company the terms of reimbursement are clearly spelled out. The insurance company will reimburse a specified percentage of a specific fee guide, less deductibles, up to a given annual limit. For example, suppose you work for ABC Widgets Ltd., which has signed a contract with We Cover All Insurance Co. The contract states that you are covered for all basic procedures at one hundred percent of the 1989 Ontario suggested fee guide. Your annual deductible is twenty-five dollars and your annual limit is $1000. You come to my office and receive fillings totalling one hundred dollars. How much of this will be covered by We Cover All Insurance Co.?

At first glance, you might think your coverage would be for one hundred dollars less your deductible of twenty-five dollars. But that may not be correct. My fees are based on the *current* Ontario fee guide, which this year is the 1991 fee guide. Your insurance company pays according to the 1989 fee guide, which is roughly ten percent below current fees. So We Cover All Insurance Co. will reimburse you for approximately ninety percent of one hundred dollars less your deductible of twenty-five dollars for a total of sixty-five dollars — ten dollars less than you expected.

The lesson to be learned here is that the fee-guide year by which the plan pays is very important. But if your insurance company bases its reimbursement on a fee guide that is one or two years out of date, don't feel too badly. I have a number of patients who work for a major Canadian company whose coverage is fifty percent based on the 1978 fee guide. Which means they get reimbursed for about fifteen percent of their dental fees! It all depends on the contract that your employer has signed and the premiums that are deducted from your pay cheque.

If I have dental insurance, do I pay the dentist or does my insurance pay directly?

This depends on your dentist. Some dentists insist that you pay for the service and that your insurance reimburses you separately. Other dentists will allow you to assign your benefits directly to the dentist by signing in a special place on the insurance form. Then you will be billed for any difference once the insurance has paid the dentist up to the limit of your coverage.

In my office, we ask our patients to pay us directly and then they receive reimbursement from the insurance company. To facilitate this, I accept a thirty-day postdated cheque as payment. This way, you will have received your repayment from the insurance company by the time the cheque is cashed. Most dentists prefer being paid directly by patients. There are fewer accounting chores involved — but there are deeper philosophical reasons for this too. I like to feel that I am serving my patients, not some nameless insurance company. I feel that my responsibility is to my patient and that my patient's responsibility is to look after paying his or her fees. I have a direct relationship with the patient regarding treatment, fees, and all other aspects of the patient-doctor relationship. The insurance company has a relationship with the patient, not with me.

Your first office visit

Why does a dentist need my medical history?

When you arrive at a new dental office the first thing you'll be asked to do is to fill out a medical-history form. The first part of this form deals with personal information such as your name, address, telephone number, occupation, age, height, and weight. Some of these questions may seem nosey to you, but they are all important.

Take your age, for example. Changes in your mouth may be normal for your age group, but not for someone ten years younger or older. Your height and weight are important for correct dosage of some medications. Even your occupation can help explain things happening in your mouth. Tooth grinding, for example, is common among stockbrokers. And I've seen notches in the front teeth of tailors and seamstresses who bite off threads!

The second part of the form deals with your previous health history. This is very important because some medical conditions can drastically alter the mode of your dental treatment. The table on the next page lists some of the questions found in this form and the reasons for their importance.

The third part of the form asks about your dental history. When was your last visit? How frequently have you seen a dentist in the past? When was the last time you had a full set of X-rays taken? Do you have any problems with extractions or freezing? And so on. These questions help to establish a profile of your dental habits. The answers may help determine the timing of treatment best suited for you.

Records completed, you are ushered into the treatment room and seated comfortably in a large reclining chair.

QUESTIONS	THEIR SIGNIFICANCE
Do you have any history of heart trouble?	If, for example, you have angina, short early-morning appointments with minimum stress are required. Nitroglycerin tablets must be available during appointment.
Do you have hemophilia (blood clotting disorder)?	Depending on type and severity, you may need special premedication. Or, your dental work may have to be done in hospital.
Do you have a history of rheumatic fever or heart murmurs?	If you have a history of rheumatic fever or murmurs related to heart valve conditions such as mitral valve prolapse, you must take antibiotics before and after each appointment.
Are you allergic to any medications?	Your dentist must know of any allergies you have before administering freezing or other types of painkiller, or prescribing antibiotics.
Do you have high blood pressure?"	If your blood pressure is extremely high, dental treatment may have to be postponed until it is under control. Sedatives may need to be prescribed before your dental appointment if anxiety elevates your blood pressure.
Are you taking any medications?	Medications prescribed or administered during dental treatment may create adverse reactions with medications you are already taking.
Are you pregnant?	During pregnancy, only emergency X-rays are usually taken. As well, hormonal changes during this time may explain some conditions such as excessive inflammation of the gums.

The external examination

The first part of a dental examination deals with the external aspects of the head and neck. First, I observe if there are any asymmetries to your face. This is a ten-dollar word to describe whether your head and neck are similar on both sides. There are many conditions that account for these differences. Swelling of the face, growths, paralysis of facial muscles, or weakened muscles on one side of the face will cause one side of the face to look different from the other side.

Next, I feel under your jaw and around your face for any enlarged or swollen glands. These may signal an infection or disease in the area. Then I position my fingers just inside your ears and ask you to open and close your mouth. I am listening and feeling for any cracking or grinding of your joints. Such noises indicate potential problems in your joints because normal, healthy joints are quiet in operation. I will talk about joint problems in the section on TMJ Syndrome in Chapter 4.

The inside of your mouth

Your throat, cheeks, bite, and gums

Now we get to the internal part of the examination. This is where you'll hear me say "open wide" for the first of many times. The first thing I check inside your mouth are the soft tissues. These include the back of the throat, the inside of the cheeks, the tongue, the bottom of the mouth (floor), the roof of the mouth (palate), and the lips. What I am looking for here are any signs of disease, such as tumors, swelling, enlargements, scrapes from sharp tooth edges, or broken restorations (fillings, crowns, or dentures).

Next I look at your bite — how your upper and lower teeth meet and mesh when you bite together.

Then I check your gums, the foundation of all your teeth. This is a very important part of the examination. As in any construction, if the foundation is strong, anything can be built on it. Your gums are the foundation of your teeth. So I check the gums for color, consistency, and width. Then, aided by a probe marked off in millimetres, I go around each tooth and measure the amount of gum recession. (I will talk about this in greater detail in Chapter 4.) I also note the amount of plaque, tartar and bleeding present around each tooth. Finally, I record any looseness or mobility for each tooth.

Your teeth

Now we finally get to the teeth themselves. I examine each tooth, checking its state of restoration. That is, I examine the condition of the fillings or other tooth restorations. I note how sound such restorations are, whether or not they need to be replaced, or whether more extensive restoration is required. I look for signs of decay and any cracks, chips, or leakage around the present restoration. Leakage occurs when there is a space between the edge of the restoration and the tooth. This means that food, plaque, and bacteria can get into this space and cause further decay.

Leakage is only one reason why an old filling needs to be replaced. Another is what is called an overhang. An overhang may occur at the time the filling is placed into the tooth. If the filling material is not properly confined within the tooth, an excess of this material hangs over the edge of the tooth at gum level. This creates an area that is difficult to clean and that traps food and bacteria. Tooth decay and gum damage may occur in the area if the problem is not corrected. Another reason for filling replacement is an open contact. This occurs when there is a space between the fillings on adjacent teeth (the filling was not extended far enough to tightly meet the adjacent tooth surface). Food gets caught in this space and it is difficult to keep clean. Eventually tooth decay and gum problems develop in loose contact areas.

Next, I tap gently on each tooth, one by one, and ask my patient to report any sensitivity. If a tooth is sensitive to tapping, it may have an inflamed area around or underneath it. This can happen when a tooth is abscessed or when a tooth carries too heavy a bite load.

X-rays

Why do I need X-rays of my teeth?

● **X-rays give a complete picture.**
To obtain a complete picture of your teeth and supporting bones, dentists must take X-rays. If dentists rely on a visual examination alone without taking X-rays, they can detect decay only on the biting surface of the teeth. This is inadequate because most tooth decay occurs in-between teeth. Unless such decay becomes very large, it cannot be seen visually.

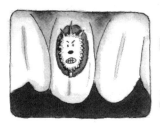 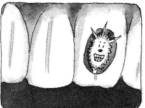 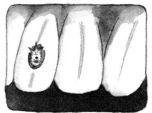

Only X-rays can detect early cavities in-between teeth. What we call secondary decay — decay under an existing filling — only shows up on X-rays. And if a filling is old and needs to be replaced, an X-ray will tell us how deep the filling is and whether the nerve of the tooth is affected.

● **X-rays show nerve canals.**
X-rays show the condition of the nerve chamber inside the tooth. Unusually large or unusually small chambers may indicate disease in the nerve chamber of that tooth.

● **X-rays show abscessed teeth.**
Small circles of pus attached to the end of a tooth's root are a sign of an abscessed tooth. X-rays can show these small circles before any pain is caused from the abscess. Treating an abscessed tooth before it becomes painful saves a lot of grief and agony.

● **X-rays show supporting bone.**

X-rays are very important checks on the health of the bone housing the roots of the teeth. X-rays will show any drop in the bone level around specific teeth. They will also show any correctable defects in the bone surrounding the teeth. Any cysts or tumors of the bone will be visible on the X-rays as well.

Sometimes the presence of extra teeth (over and above the usual number), which have not yet grown through, can be seen on X-rays. Conversely, X-rays in children can show that some permanent teeth are congenitally missing. That means that they simply never formed. Knowing this in advance allows the dentist to plan for any future replacement of these teeth. In growing children, X-rays clearly show whether all permanent teeth are developing normally. The location and position of unerupted wisdom teeth can be seen only on X-rays.

These are some of the many good reasons why dental X-rays are a must.

What about the dangers of radiation?

We dentists take great care to ensure that our patients' radiation exposure is minimal. We achieve this in several ways. First, we cover the body with a lead-lined apron. This protects all the organs, most importantly the reproductive organs. Most dentists now use a lead collar on the lead apron, to protect the thymus and thyroid glands, too.

Next, we use a long cone on the X-ray machine itself. This cone produces a very narrow, small radiation area that can be focussed on specific teeth. It also moves the X-ray head further away from the patient. As well, the film we use has lead lining on one side of it. This means that once the X-rays reach the film, they are not allowed to go any further but are absorbed by the lead lining instead. Finally, we use a very fast film for dental X-rays. This means that very little radiation is required to expose the film, again greatly reducing patient exposure.

Dental X-rays are safe.

Recently, the Ontario Dental Association released a chart comparing the different amounts of X-ray exposure for different types of medical X-rays. Here is an excerpt from that table*:

HIGH DOSE GROUP	UNITS OF RADIATION
Barium enema (lower G.I. series)	875
Mammography: breast examination (exposure per breast)	500
Small bowel series	422
MEDIUM DOSE GROUP	
Gall bladder	168
Pelvis	133
Hip	72
LOW DOSE GROUP	
Femur (upper leg)	21
Dental (whole mouth)	9

* Excerpted with permission from the Ontario Dental Association's *Health Hazards Manual, 1989.*

The chart clearly shows that the amount of radiation from a dental series is a fraction of that from any other procedure. **Dental X-rays are safe.**

In a standard dental X-ray series, we take sixteen films. This is necessary to show at least two views of each tooth. Sometimes a shadow of another tooth may look like a problem area on a particular film. Looking at that same area from another angle on the next film will show the dentist whether or not there really is a problem.

Can I refuse to have dental X-rays?

Dental X-rays are one of the most important sources of
information about your teeth and supporting structures
that your dentist has. So I try to dissuade the occasional
patients who categorically refuse to have any X-rays. I try to
make them understand that dental X-rays *are* safe. I carefully explain the limitations patients impose on me by
refusing X-rays. In the face of absolute refusal of the patient
to have X-rays, I will perform only the most basic treatment
necessary, such as small fillings and cleanings. I will not
undertake any extractions, root canals, or involved reconstructive treatment. And for my own records and protec-
tion, I ask those patients to sign a form saying that they
understand that by not allowing any X-rays, they relieve me
of any responsibility for not treating conditions evident only
on X-rays. Most patients change their minds when we get to
this stage. They realize that this is serious business and that
taking X-rays is in their interest.

Taking models of your teeth

If I note that the examination or X-rays show missing teeth,
damaged teeth, teeth that are badly ground down, or teeth
that mesh poorly between the upper and lower jaw, I will
take models of your teeth. This is completely painless. I mix
a jelly-like solution in a tray and place one part over your
top teeth and one part over your bottom teeth. Once these
molds are taken, I ask you to bite into some wax to make a
record of how your upper and lower teeth meet. Then my
assistant pours a plaster material into the molds and voilà
we have a plaster model of your mouth. Models are very
useful for judging whether sufficient space is present for
restoring teeth. It gives us a three-dimensional model of the
position and angle of each tooth and it is invaluable when
designing dentures, bridges, implants, and the like.

To recap: Your first visit consists of an examination X-
rays, and, if necessary, the making of models of your teeth.
Now we can go on to visit two: the consultation
appointment.

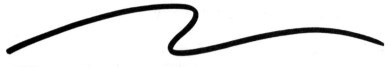

The consultation appointment

This appointment may be very short if, after analyzing your X-rays, examination findings, and models, I find that everything appears to be OK. But if I find that extensive treatment is required, this appointment may last an hour or more. I usually conduct my consultation appointments away from the treatment room. There is a special consultation room where we can sit at a table and go over all the findings in a relaxed setting.

Planning your treatment

I usually divide the treatment plan into phases. Urgent procedures are planned first, of course. They include things such as extractions, root-canal treatments, abscessed teeth, treatment of severe gum problems, and cleaning and filling decayed teeth.

Phase two is the stabilizing phase. This includes more extensive restorations of teeth, more gradual treatments to bring the gums back to optimum health, and other treatments that help you to maintain a healthy mouth.

The third phase is the reconstructive phase. This phase includes replacing missing teeth, rebuilding your bite, and improving the functioning and cosmetics of your mouth.

At each stage, I will tell you precisely what needs to be done. I will describe the treatment as clearly and simply as possible; I will tell you what it will cost and how much time it will take. Then we will agree on a timetable to complete each phase of treatment. If time or finances are a problem, we will discuss alternatives to the proposed treatment plan. Once we both agree on a treatment, timing, and payment plan, we can schedule appointments. I firmly believe that taking unhurried time — up-front — is crucial to an amicable dentist-patient relationship. I strongly recommend finding a dentist who agrees with this approach.

Changing bad habits

A complex reconstructive treatment plan may take several years to complete. But often what takes the longest is re-learning how to view and care for your mouth. A mouth that requires a lot of treatment is likely to be a mouth that has been neglected for a long time. It requires a change of habits and attitudes on the part of the patient to correct this problem. A lot of time, money, and effort spent reconstructing a mouth is useless if it will be neglected again. Dental treatment is a cooperative affair between the patient and the dentist.

Dental cleanings

Dental cleanings are very important because they help maintain the health of your gums. Your gums are the foundation of your teeth. Just like a house, strong teeth require a strong foundation.

Regular six-month cleanings

Some people take such excellent care of their teeth and gums that my office sees them only once a year for cleanings. But these people are the exceptions. Most people who take meticulous care of their gums and teeth at home, who floss and brush daily, require a regular six-month cleaning by a dentist or dental hygienist to keep their gums and teeth healthy.

A dentist or a hygienist?

Either your dentist or a hygienist may clean your teeth. Both are fully qualified and capable. In my office, hygienists do all the cleanings. My attitude is that they are the specialists for this job. Hygienists clean teeth all day, every day. They have a great deal of practice and experience, so they're the true experts. But we dentists are trained to clean teeth, too and many dentists prefer to do their own cleanings.

What actually happens during a cleaning?

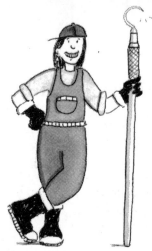

The main goal of a dental cleaning is to remove hardened, caked-on plaque. This hardened material is called **calculus** or **tartar.** When you brush your teeth at home you are only removing soft plaque. This is why (as I explained in Chapter 1), you don't scrub your teeth. To remove hardened calculus, the hygienist uses special sharp and angled instruments called **scalers**. Scalers are applied or hooked under the ledge of the calculus and on the side of your tooth. The calculus is removed from the tooth with an upward motion. The hygienist carefully traces each surface of the tooth and scales it to ensure that no calculus is left behind. Once all teeth are calculus-free, they are polished with paste on a rubber cup. The rubber cup rotates on the end of a handpiece or drill, rubbing the abrasive paste onto the tooth and smoothing out areas where there was calculus before the scaling. This polishing also removes any stains and spots from the teeth and leaves them smooth, shiny and clean. When you run your tongue against your teeth after a professional cleaning, you'll find that they feel great!

Do cleanings hurt?

If you have regular cleanings and if you look after your teeth at home in-between visits, there should be very little calculus present on your teeth. This means that very little scaling will be needed and most of the cleaning appointment will be spent on polishing. Such appointments are very pleasant and relaxing. You can actually look forward to them. But if your visits are irregular and you don't practice proper oral hygiene at home, you can be sure you will have a great deal of calculus and plaque on your teeth and that a lot of scaling will be required. This is the less comfortable part of the appointment. As well, all that calculus and plaque will inflame your gums. Inflamed gums are much more sensitive and tender than firm healthy ones. So a professional cleaning may be uncomfortable under these circumstances.

The bottom line is this: Some hygienists are more gentle than others. And some patients have a very low pain threshold. What may be agony to some is a piece of cake to others. So here is my advice: If your cleaning is really uncomfortable, tell your dentist. If ninety percent of the healthy patients find regular cleanings painful, it may be time for the dentist to have a chat with the hygienist. On the other hand, if you are the first to complain, you may be unusually sensitive. There is no need to be ashamed. What you may need is a little freezing before the scaling. Or maybe you should request the use of laughing gas during your scaling. Lots of my patients use laughing gas when they're having their teeth cleaned. In fact, my wife will only have cleanings done with laughing gas. Yet I still love her.

Fluorides

Many dentists will recommend a fluoride treatment after a scaling and polishing. When I tell new patients this, they often question the need for fluoride. After all, isn't it just for kids?

Not any more. We used to recommend fluoride for children up to the age of eighteen or so because they are in the cavity-prone years and using fluoride is an excellent way to strengthen teeth against the ravages of tooth decay. Fluoride works by binding to tooth surfaces. These surfaces are then better able to resist the acidic onslaught of plaque. This means less decay.

Two additional reasons adults should use fluorides

In addition to strengthening your teeth against regular cavities, fluorides have been shown in research to have two important new uses. First, they inhibit the growth of the type of bacteria responsible for periodontal (gum) disease.

This means that fluoride applications can help fight peri-odontal disease, which is found mostly (though not exclu-sively), in adults.

Second, fluorides also help prevent a special type of decay known as **root caries**. Root caries are cavities or decay in the root portion of the tooth, below the gum. These are different from regular cavities that occur in the crown portion of the tooth, above the gum line. Root caries occur in people whose gums have receded or moved down the side of the root due to periodontal disease. They are very difficult to treat since it is often difficult for the dentist to get in-between the roots of back teeth in order to fill them. We will talk more about root caries in Chapter 4. For now, suffice it to say that fluorides help prevent root caries.

Fluoride treatments are usually done using a foam tray. This tray looks like two letter U's. One of the U's fits over your bottom teeth, the other over the top ones. You bite into these trays and hold them there for two to four min-utes. Many gel flavors are available. Champagne, pina colada, and butterscotch are the adult flavors of choice in our office.

Should I use a fluoride rinse or gel at home?

Ask your dentist if using a fluoride rinse or gel at home is recommended. Fluoride treatments are effective in the office because they are applied right after scaling and polishing, before saliva and plaque get a chance to coat your teeth. This means that the fluoride gets into close contact with your teeth and there are fewer bacteria for it to act upon. At home, where your teeth may not be as per-fectly clean, a rinse may be less effective. However, if you have ongoing periodontal disease or a lot of recurrent root caries, you may find weekly or even daily applications of fluoride gels or rinses helpful. Ask your dentist what is best for you.

In our office, we have made special plastic trays for a number of our patients to use with fluoride gels at home. Many of these patients' periodontal health has improved dramatically. Others have had a marked reduction in cavities.

Fluoridated water

Most cities and towns now have fluoridated water, which provides enough oral intake. If you do not have fluoridated water or if the fluoride concentration in your drinking water is less than 1.0 ppm (parts per million), you can call your local water authority to find out if the water you are drinking contains fluoride.

Fluoride is also found naturally in some well water. If you are using well water, you can have it tested for fluoride content.

Fluoride ingested through drinking fluoridated water is especially beneficial for growing children. It is incorporated into the child's forming tooth enamel and makes the child's teeth much more resistant to decay. Fluoride ingested through fluoridated drinking water also benefits adult teeth, through its presence in the saliva and gums. Some studies suggest that the teeth, bathed in fluoride, are strengthened against cavities.

Fluoride supplements

If you find that your water supply is not fluoridated or that it contains less than 1.0 ppm of fluoride, you may want to consult your dentist regarding the use of fluoride tablet supplements. The following table illustrates suggested dosages for persons over the age of three years.

Amount of fluoride in water (ppm)	Sodium fluoride (mg)	Fluoride (mg)
0	2.2	1.0
0.2	1.8	0.8
0.4	1.3	0.6
0.6	0.9	0.4

For children two to three years of age, the doses should be reduced by half. For children two months to two years, 0.5 mg of sodium fluoride may be administered in drops.

Be sure to consult with your dentist before taking fluoride supplements.

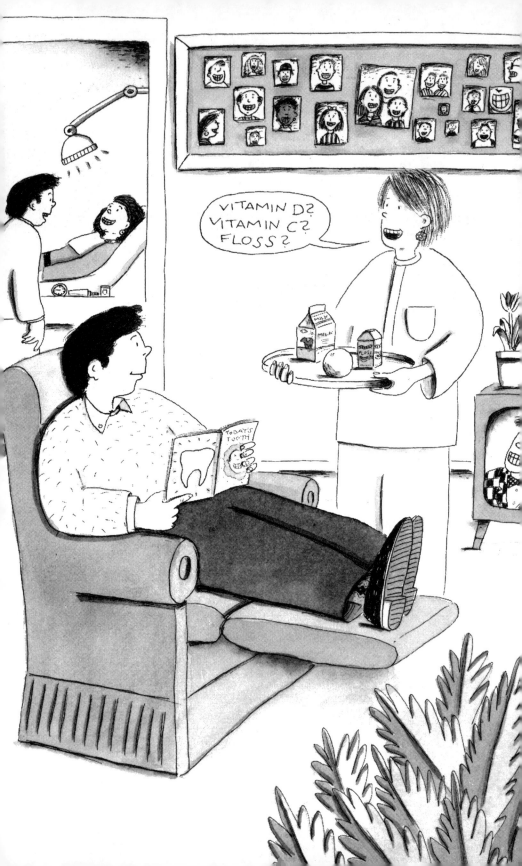

Your dentist and the tools of the trade

A dentist's office can be a strange and threatening environment. But once you know what's what in it, you won't be a bit worried. I promise! So let's go on a guided tour of a dental office.

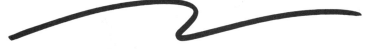

Your dentist's office

A new kind of reception room

If you haven't been to a dentist in a while, you're in for a surprise. Most modern dental offices have done away with what was known as The Waiting Room — the small, cramped room filled with plain chairs and a few torn, outdated magazines. Now we call the entrance area the reception room and it looks very different. The small wicket-window with a curt receptionist behind it saying "Next!", is gone. The room is usually an airy, open-concept space done in

bright colors with sofas, couches, or armchairs instead of
the line-up of straight-backed chairs in the waiting room of
yore. In my office, we have done away with the reception
counter altogether and replaced it with a small desk where
a receptionist sits. The idea is to make you feel comfortable •
and at home as soon as you come in. The living-room
atmosphere creates a relaxed mood for the patient, and
having the receptionist at eye-level allows for easy
communication.

And, thanks to a large increase over the last two decades
in the number of dentists in North America, you probably
won't be kept waiting long. Dentists don't overbook much
anymore. They know their patients are busy people who can
take their mouths down the block if they're not happy.

Most dental offices are computerized now. This makes
financial dealings clearer and faster and means fewer errors
with your account. Most dental computers can print up
your insurance forms on the spot, which speeds up your
insurance reimbursements. And in some areas of Canada
and the United States, insurance companies are hooked up
directly to these computers, making things move even more
quickly.

Become familiar with the treatment room.

The modern treatment room, where your dentist examines
and treats you, is designed for comfort and relaxation. Most
newer offices follow the open-concept design, with walls
only six to seven feet high, and an open space between the
top of the wall and the ceiling. This gives the treatment
room an airy feeling and prevents patients from feeling
confined or constrained. These days, the only place you'll
find dental treatment being done behind closed doors and
accompanied by muffled screams is in a theatre specializing
in old movies. Modern dentistry is very nearly painless and
needs no doors.

In the middle of the room is the dental chair. This too
has changed over the years. Dentists used to work standing
up while the patient sat upright. Some older dentists still

practise this way. Chiropractors and back specialists can instantly spot an X-ray of an old-style dentist's back. It has an S-shaped curve developed from the dentists attempts to peer into people's mouths from the side and upside down.

Now dentists sit down to do their work and patients lie fully reclined. The patient chairs of today are unbelievably comfortable. In my office, not a day goes by without at least one patient wishing for a similar chair at home in which to read or watch TV. Because they sit over the patient's mouth, dentists' backs and limbs are not as strained and they can work faster and more efficiently. They can accomplish more at each appointment and need fewer appointments with the patient to complete the dental work.

The dental assistant sits at the head of the patient, across from the dentist, in order to see directly into the patient's mouth. The assistant then sees exactly what is being done and knows what instruments or materials to hand the dentist next. This type of arrangement is referred to as four-handed dentistry, because both the assistant and the dentist work on the patient's mouth at the same time.

Now let's look at some of the more common instruments and pieces of equipment used by dentists and their assistants.

The dental light

The mouth is a dark, confined space and proper illumination is essential during a dental procedure. A proper dental light delivers bright, focused light into the mouth and minimizes shadows cast by dentists' hands or instruments. Because the light is so well focused, none of it shines in the patient's eyes, and the patient remains more relaxed.

The dental unit

The dental unit consists of a small **utility tray, dental handpieces (drills)**, and an **air-water syringe**. This unit is the heart of a dental operatory.

The location of the dental unit has changed over the years and dentists still can't agree on the best place for it. In the past, the dental unit swung on an extension arm over the patient. Because dentists at that time worked unassisted, the utility tray was large enough to hold all instruments and materials within easy reach. As more dentists began using assistants who handed instruments to them, dentists became less reliant on a utility tray. However, they still needed the handpieces in easy reach.

Nowadays several placements of the dental unit are used. These include placement over the patient as in the past, (but now the patient is lying down); off to the side of the dental chair on the dentist's side; or behind the patient's head. The latter two systems have the advantage of being hidden from the patient's view. Most patients cringe at the immediate sight of the "drills" — patients are better able to relax when that equipment is out of view.

Call it a shaper, not a drill.

The main parts of the dental unit are the slow- and high-speed handpieces. We dentists do anything to avoid calling these instruments "drills." I like to call them "cleaners" and "shapers" because that is what they do. You see, handpieces don't actually drill holes. If you come in with a cavity to be filled, you already have the hole. I don't need to drill it for you. I clean the cavity by removing soft decayed matter. I shape it so that the filling material will stay in place for a long time. But I don't drill a hole. You supply that. So don't ever think of the handpieces as drills again! Shapers, cleaners, smoothers, or Mr. Buzz-Buzz sound so much better, wouldn't you agree?

Modern handpieces are air-driven turbines. This means that high-pressure air delivered by plastic hoses rotates a small propeller inside the handpiece. This provides the spinning motion for the shaping inserts to clean and shape cavities. The high-speed handpieces rotate at speeds of 400,000 rpm. Compare this to the original handpieces at the turn of the century which were driven by the dentist's foot, and you quickly understand why dentistry is painless today. The higher speed of the tooth preparation and the diminished level of vibration provide increased comfort. These high-speed handpieces also emit a constant water spray to keep the tooth from overheating as it is shaped and cleaned. Most of the newer handpieces come with built-in lights which greatly enhance visibility in those hard-to-reach and hard-to-see areas. They are a blessing to a dentist's strained eyes.

The slow-speed handpiece is used primarily for polishing and smoothing of restorations. But as newer materials become available, it is being used less and less.

The air-water syringe is used for flushing out, cleaning, rinsing, and drying prepared teeth. Many of the newer bonding materials demand an absolutely dry tooth surface for proper bond formation.

Suction

The assistant usually controls the suction, which removes the water from your mouth during the shaping and cleaning process of tooth preparation. It also takes away any excess debris or filling materials from inside your mouth. Newer suctions are much stronger than the straw-like saliva ejectors that older dentists hooked onto your lip. Those were designed simply to remove the saliva from your mouth.

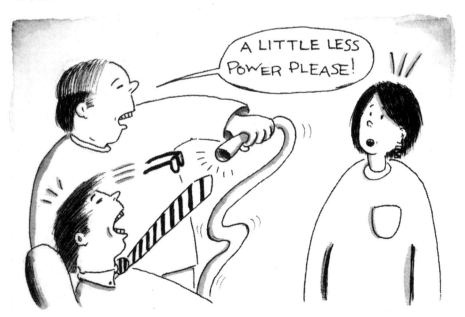

X-ray machine

X-ray units are now small and lightweight. This change allows for greater manoeuvrability and for precision of placement and aim. Most X-ray units are equipped with a long cone which focuses the X-rays on a small area, limiting a patient's exposure to the rays as much as possible.

Curing light units

These are fairly recent additions to a dentist's arsenal. Most of the newer generation of white and bonded filling materials are cured (hardened) by exposure to visible light. Fifteen years ago, these lights were usually ultraviolet. But concerns about the negative effects of ultraviolet light on dental staffs' eyesight have resulted in the development of materials that harden under high-intensity visible light. Even this kind of light poses dangers, however. As dentists shine the curing light on patients' new fillings, they will place a dark orange shield between their own eyes and the light. Current research indicates that repeated exposure of the dentist's eyes to this high-intensity light causes premature aging of the retina of the eye.

The amalgamator

The amalgamator mixes silver amalgam fillings (I discuss the controversy about silver amalgam fillings in Chapter 4, pages 80–83). These are made of a mixture of mercury and silver with small quantities of other substances, such as copper. The mercury must be thoroughly mixed with the silver for the combination to create an effective filling. Dentists used to use a mortar and pestle to mix these two substances. I still remember my first dentist doing this. Now high-speed mixing machines or amalgamators do the job more quickly and efficiently. Most of these machines are quite noisy and make that characteristic whirring noise you hear just before your tooth is filled.

Laughing gas: mask and equipment

I will discuss laughing gas itself later in this chapter. The gas is delivered to the patient either by a portable cart which contains the oxygen and nitrous oxide (laughing gas) tanks or through a built-in system. In the latter case, the tanks are kept in a separate storage room and pipes in the walls carry the gas to the patient's chair. The only part of this equipment that the patient actually sees is the mask that fits over the nose. There are different kinds of masks available. Most dentists use a hood-type mask, which catches the air the patient breathes out and removes it from the room. This is because the air breathed out contains laughing gas and if the patient exhales it straight out, the people in the room may get some too. I doubt that most patients would want a slightly "buzzed" dentist working in their mouths!

Root canal file sterilizer
This is a small electrical appliance. It keeps a container of salt at a very high temperature. During a root canal procedure, files and instruments are dipped into this hot salt for ten to fifteen seconds killing any bacteria on them and making them clean and sterile.

Carpule warmer
This piece of equipment uses a small lightbulb to warm up **anesthetic carpules** (freezings) to body temperature. Warmed-up freezings may sound contradictory but in fact they are much more comfortable to the patient than cold or room-temperature solutions.

Ultrasonic cleaner
This is used mostly by the hygienist. It has a handle just like a dental handpiece, but at the end of it there is a stationary probe or scaler. Instead of spinning, it vibrates at very high frequencies. When this instrument is brought in contact with the calculus (tartar) on the teeth, its vibrations knock the tartar off the tooth. As with the handpiece, a steady stream of water comes out of this instrument at all times. This water cools the probe, which otherwise would heat up tremendously from the vibrations.

I hope that knowing a bit more about your dentist's equipment makes you more comfortable. If nothing else, I hope you come away from this discussion never thinking of the "D" word again. Remember, the handpiece cleans and shapes your teeth. There is no "D-ing" involved — ever!

Dentistry without pain

How painless dentistry has become ... painless

According to statistics, fifty percent of the population see a dentist on an emergency basis only. One out of two people! It doesn't take a genius to figure out why this is so. It's called "fear of pain." Many adults remember terrifying visits to the dentist as children. Often they were primed by horror stories told to them by their parents, who learned their fears from *their* parents. Just about everybody has heard some awful story about a vicious dentist inflicting agonizing pain on a hapless victim.

Where did all these notions come from? Well, in the old days, dentistry *could* be unpleasant. And everything is bigger and scarier for children. Once these memories set in, they can linger for a long time. Sometimes I think everyone thinks of dentists as similar to the cruel and sadistic character played by Steve Martin in the classic horror comedy, "Little Shop of Horrors."

Dental phobia has nothing to do with courage. Picture the following scene: A six-foot-four, 220-pound policeman comes into my office. He folds himself into my dental chair. He is so tall his head sticks out three inches over the edge of the chair and his feet are almost in the next room.

Now I don't know how you feel about policemen, but I think they require exceptional courage to wear a badge in today's violent world. But this six-foot-four bruiser, who thinks nothing of kicking his way into crack houses and confronting armed drug addicts in dark alleyways, is trembling in my dental chair, terrified of the needle I am about to use to freeze his mouth!

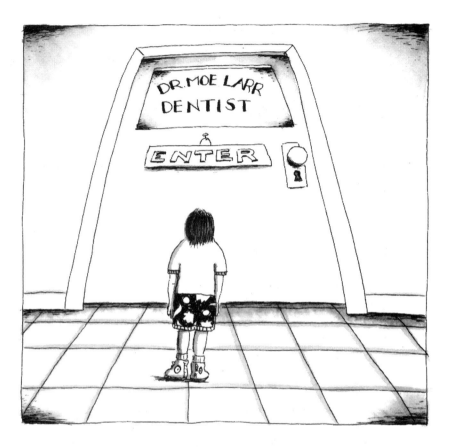

Is he a coward? Hardly. It's just that somewhere along the way, some experience, conversation, or perception of dental discomfort stuck in his memory — and grew out of proportion in his imagination. Now every time he thinks of a dentist he breaks out in a cold sweat.

You see, fear of dentists plays no favorites. Whether you're big or small, brave or not so brave, a crane-operator or a librarian, you can learn to love your dentist and never be afraid of a dental visit again.

Scout's honor.

How can I make this promise? Simple. Modern dentistry is so sophisticated that the smallest discomfort in the dental chair has become a thing of the past. So let's go down the list of pain-free techniques.

Pain-free Technique #1: freezing by injection

The oldest and most common method of anesthetizing (freezing) a tooth is with an injection. Before you cringe, wait a moment: there have been some great advances in freezing.

● Before you see anything resembling a needle, your gums are painted with an anesthetic paste. This paste numbs the top few layers of tissue, so you don't feel even the slightest initial prick of the needle.

● We use disposable needles. You are assured of a sterilized needle every time. And of equal importance, you are assured of a perfectly sharp needle.

● Anesthetic solutions have changed for the better. Novocaine is gone and it's been replaced with a myriad of fast-acting solutions that are more effective and have fewer unpleasant consequences. This means that only three to five minutes after the anesthetic is placed, your tooth is completely numb.

But what if the very thought of needles terrifes me?

Pain-free Technique #2: laughing gas

Laughing gas (nitrous oxide) may be the answer for you if you can't bear the sight of a needle. Laughing gas will give you a sensation of euphoria and detachment. It won't put you to sleep. You are awake and fully aware of your environment, yet you're completely uninterested in what's going on. It's a bit like having a stiff drink or two. Does that sound like your idea of the perfect dental appointment? That's not all laughing gas does. Nitrous oxide seems to affect the perception of time so the appointment seems shorter to you than it actually is. And it has some amnesiac effects too, so you may not be able to recall many details of your dental appointment. Could you possibly ask for more?

Are there any dangers in using laughing gas?

In the early part of the twentieth century, laughing gas was a favourite gag at parties. A canister of the gas would be released in a room, making the partygoers feel pleasantly giddy.

Nowadays nitrous oxide is restricted to professional use because if it is used undiluted and in excessive doses, it can be fatal. But don't worry. Dentists and doctors use it only in carefully controlled combinations, in conjunction with oxygen. No more than sixty percent nitrous oxide to forty percent oxygen is used. Most people require no more than twenty-five to thirty-five percent concentrations of the gas to achieve the desired effect.

Can anyone use laughing gas safely?
Almost everyone is a candidate for nitrous oxide sedation. It's especially effective for children too young to sit still for an injection. Pregnant women are advised not to use it during the first three months of their pregnancy but they can use it after that.

How laughing gas works
Laughing gas works very quickly. Five to ten minutes into the appointment, the patient feels comfortable and mellow. When the dentist has completed the work he or she stops the nitrous oxide gas and gives the patient a breath of pure oxygen gas to bring him or her back to reality. The effects of the laughing gas are "washed off" after ten to fifteen minutes of pure oxygen. However, the patient may still feel a bit groggy and driving is not recommend for a few hours afterward.

Pain-free Technique #3: pre-appointment sedation
Pre-appointment sedation involves the use of tranquilizers or sedatives prior to the dental appointment. These may be taken orally several hours before the appointment or injected intramuscularly by the dentist just before the appointment. This area of dental sedation is very individual-ized. Only your dentist, after reviewing your medical history and your concerns about your dental appointment, can prescribe oral medications for your particular needs. I prescribe medication such as this only for excessively nervous or stressed patients. One reason I am very careful is that some of these medications can cause drug dependence.

It is absolutely imperative to use these kinds of medication exactly as prescribed by your dentist or physician. Never mix them with other prescription drugs or with alcohol.

Pain-free Technique #4: hypnosis

Every major city has several dentists who practise medical hypnosis. I am not talking here about vaudeville-act trances. You won't walk or quack like a duck during your appointments. I am talking about a medically-induced state of mind that does work for some patients. The dental work is usually preceded by one or two appointments during which the dentist-hypnotist practises putting you into a hypnotic state. You will become accustomed to being totally relaxed, and to entering and coming out of the hypnotic state. Once you've mastered this, you set up a dental appointment. There the dentist-hypnotist quickly leads you into the hypnotic state by using specific words and phrases. During the initial appointments, the dentist-hypnotist has conditioned you to relax, to breathe regularly, to feel no anxiety, and to trust that you will feel absolutely no discomfort. Once the dental work is done, you again follow a predetermined set of commands to exit from the hypnotic state. Often the dentist will insert an instruction, during your hypnotic state, to forget the entire appointment (all, that is, except paying the bill!). Dental hypnosis is a legitimate means of reducing the anxiety of a dental appointment and of helping patients relax. If you are interested in this mode of sedation, contact your local dental society. It will have a listing of area dentists who use hypnosis.

Pain-free Technique #5: acupuncture

A few North American dentists use acupuncture to reduce any sensations of pain or discomfort during a dental procedure. Acupuncture has been used in China and other parts of the Far East for thousands of years. Traditional acupuncture involves inserting long, thin needles into specific parts of the body such as the lower arm, hand, and earlobes to block the transmission of pain messages to the brain. There are several theories as to why this works. The most widely

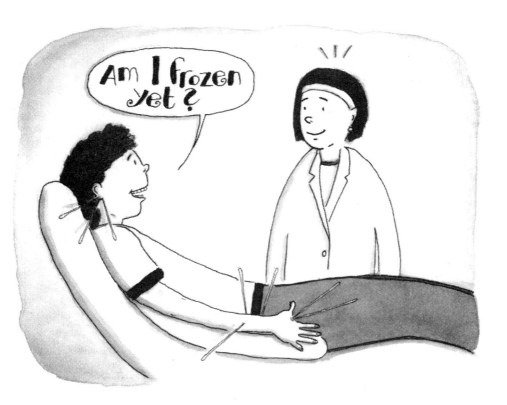

accepted ones cite the release of endorphins (natural pain-killing substances in the body) in sites related to pain.

Although we often see films of patients in China undergoing major surgeries such as appendectomies or gall bladder removals using only acupuncture anesthesia, we see fairly few followers of this practice in North America. My belief is that patients who are afraid of needles would prefer a single, quick, standard freezing to several long acupuncture needles in their arm or earlobes. However, this is not always the case because some dentists practise this form of anesthesia with great success.

Pain-free Technique #6: intravenous sedation

Intravenous sedation is often used for complex extractions such as wisdom teeth. Sedative drugs such as Valium are introduced into the arm of the patient through an intravenous injection. The patient quickly becomes heavily sedated although not completely unconscious. The patient remains groggy for several hours and must be accompanied home by a responsible adult.

This type of sedation may be administered only by certain qualified dentists. All oral surgeons are qualified to administer it, as are some other dentist-specialists who have done additional training and earned a degree in anesthesia. Any dentist who has completed a certified course in intravenous sedation may administer this form of sedation as well. I will talk about oral surgeons later on, but here I would like to make a distinction between oral surgeons and dental surgeons. Every dentist is a dental surgeon. This is because dentists are qualified to perform procedures on live tissues such as teeth and gums. Oral surgeons, on the other hand, are dentists who have undergone an additional four to five years of training. They are trained in procedures dealing with the bones of the mouth and surrounding tissues. Their areas of expertise range from the complicated removal of oddly positioned teeth to rebuilding jaws and mouths. They are also trained in heavy sedative procedures, and general anesthesia enabling them to perform these procedures.

Pain-free Technique #7: general anesthesia

General anesthesia is sometimes recommended for major procedures such as impacted wisdom-tooth extractions, or for people who, for whatever reason, cannot tolerate any dental treatment using simpler modes of sedation.

General anesthesia, or GA for short, is what is commonly referred to as being "put out" or "put to sleep." It is administered intravenously and is very powerful. Patients under GA are unconscious and unable to protect their breathing pathways or airways. So a tube must be inserted into their windpipes to deliver oxygen to the lungs. As well, all other vital signs such as the heartbeat must be closely monitored. GA is usually performed in a hospital setting. However, GA may be performed in a dental office if proper staff and emergency equipment are available. Only qualified dentist-anesthetists or oral surgeons may perform this procedure.

A dentist without specialized training in anesthesia can use GA only if a qualified anesthetist and support staff are present in the office. Qualified "travelling" anesthetists are available. So if you require this type of sedation and want your own dentist to perform the work, you can have your dentist arrange for one of these mobile anesthetists to come to the office for your appointment.

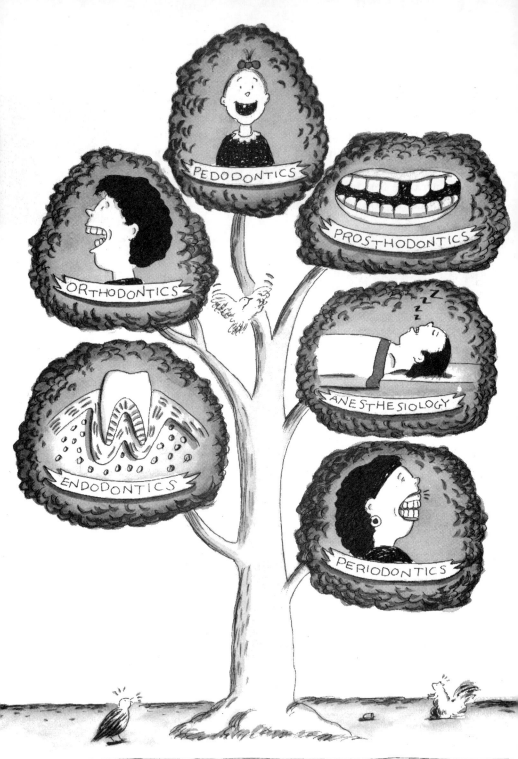

DENTIST TREE—DENTISTUS VARIETUS

The many branches of dentistry

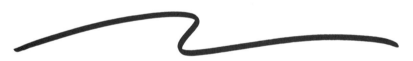

General practitioners and specialists

Your family dentist is a general practitioner (G.P.) of dentistry. The official degree is Doctor of Dental Surgery, or D.D.S. A general practitioner in dentistry is similar to a medical general practitioner or family doctor. They both have a general knowledge of the entire field in their discipline. If you come to your physician with a particularly difficult heart problem, you are referred to a specialist in heart conditions, normally a cardiologist. It is the same in dentistry. If you come to me, a general practitioner in dentistry, with a badly impacted wisdom tooth, you will be referred to an oral surgeon, a specialist in the field of wisdom teeth.

Just as you can be referred to a myriad of medical specialists, you can also be referred to various dental specialists when your family dentist feels you would benefit from their expertise.

However, family dentists are trained in all aspects of dentistry and, since they are all individuals, they all have different talents, likes, and dislikes. Some dentists may have a particular knack for extracting impacted wisdom teeth. They may like the challenge, they may have had a lot of experience with such extractions, or they may have taken additional courses of study in the subject. Such dentists would only refer extremely unusual cases to an oral surgeon. Other G.P.'s may dislike extractions. Their strengths may be in cosmetic dentistry. So they would probably refer even the simplest extractions to an oral surgeon. You may or may not be referred to a dental specialist, depending on your dentist's skills and preferences, and on the severity of your particular condition.

The specialists

A specialist in dentistry is a person who first became a general dentist and then underwent one to four years of additional training in his or her chosen field of interest.

Once dentists become specialists and hang out shingles announcing their area of expertise, they usually limit their practices to that particular area. Not many periodontists (gum specialists) will do your fillings for you.

Here is a list of dental specialists.

The endodontist	A specialist in root canal treatments. The endodontist usually handles cases where access to the nerve canals of the tooth is very difficult.
The orthodontist	A specialist in straightening teeth and correcting bite problems. Orthodontists see both children and adults.

The pedodontist	A specialist in the treatment of children. This specialist is an expert in managing a child during a dental visit, as well as in the unique problems of growth and development of the mouth.
The periodontist	A specialist in treatment of gum disease. Periodontists also do the lion's share of gum surgery in dentistry.
The prosthodontist	A specialist in replacing missing teeth with bridges, dentures, or implants. Prosthodontists are the specialists who tackle full reconstructions of badly deteriorated mouths.
The oral or maxillo-facial surgeon	A specialist in rebuilding bony sections of the mouth and face which need treatment as a result of accidents or birth defects. The oral surgeon performs any corrective bone surgery of the jaws and any extractions of difficult teeth, especially wisdom teeth. This surgeon is qualified to perform these procedures using heavy sedation techniques.
The anesthesiologist	A general practitioner who is trained to administer heavy sedation methods during dental treatment.

In the following sections I will discuss each area of dentistry, and outline the situations where your dentist may want to refer you to a specialist in that field.

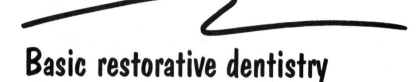

Basic restorative dentistry

Basic, garden-variety dentistry is called **restorative dentistry.** Essentially this means the filling of cavities and restoring of teeth to their original form and function.

To understand what a cavity is and how it forms we must first look at the components of a tooth.

What's a tooth made of?

A tooth is divided into two main parts — the **crown** and the **root**. The crown is the part that's above the gum. It's what you see when you look at teeth in a healthy mouth. The root is the part of the tooth embedded in the jawbone and covered by your gums. If we were to cut the whole tooth (crown and root) down the middle, along its long axis, we would see that the tooth is made up of four components. The bulk of the tooth, crown, and root is made of **dentin**. Dentin is a hard, bone-like, yellow material. It is actually a little harder than bone and it is composed of a multitude of tiny tubules. These can be properly seen only under a microscope.

In the root portion of the tooth, the dentin is hollow. This hollow part is shaped like a canal or a long, narrow funnel. In the crown portion, the dentin has a hollowed-out space or chamber in the middle. The canals of the root and the chamber of the crown are connected. In these hollow spaces are nerves, blood, and lymphatic vessels. They enter the tooth through the tip of each root, travel up the root in the hollow canal, and fill the hollow chamber in the crown portion of the tooth. In the crown portion, the dentin is covered by a layer of material called **enamel**. Enamel is the hardest substance in our bodies. It is white, and gives teeth that characteristic whitish appearance. The root portion of dentin is covered by a thin layer of a fairly soft substance called **cementum**. Under normal conditions, cementum is embedded in the jawbone and covered by gums. Normally, the only part of the tooth exposed to the outside world is the hard enamel.

What causes a cavity?

Picture a normal posterior tooth or molar. It has a number of grooves on its chewing surface. Unless it is the last tooth, it touches two other teeth — one in front of it and one behind. Sugar snacks love to settle into these grooves, nooks, and crannies on the chewing surfaces of your back teeth and on the areas between adjacent teeth that can only be cleaned by flossing. These sugar snacks are prime feeding grounds for **bacteria** called **Streptococci mutans**, S. mutans for short.

How do S. mutans cause cavities?

Food debris, especially sugars, together with larger protein molecules from saliva and bacteria, form a whitish coating on your teeth known as **plaque**. If you don't brush your teeth for a day, you can scrape this plaque off the necks of your teeth with your fingernail. Depending on the type of food debris present, different types of bacteria will be present in the plaque. S. mutans will be present in large numbers if sugar is part of this debris. S. mutans bacteria feed on sugar and when they are finished with it, they excrete a very acidic waste product. This acid is so strong that it simply dissolves the enamel of the tooth in the area where it is excreted.

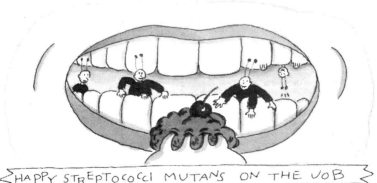

HAPPY STREPTOCOCCI MUTANS ON THE JOB

Although enamel is the hardest substance in our bodies, it dissolves as easily as ice melts in warm water when it is exposed to this acid. Once a layer of enamel has been dissolved, a small defect or cavity exists in the outer shell of the tooth. Now the plaque and the S. mutans in it have an even better place to hide to avoid both toothbrush and floss. As S. mutans eat more sugar, they produce more acid and dissolve layers of enamel deeper inside the tooth. The small original defect or cavity now becomes quite deep. This in turn provides an even better hiding place for the plaque and the bacteria. The vicious cycle continues and the cavity becomes larger and larger. Once the enamel has been dissolved right through, the underlying dentin starts to deteriorate from the acidic wastes of the S. mutans. Since dentin is softer than enamel, it dissolves even faster, creating a bigger and bigger cavity.

How cavities grow larger

A cavity starts as a small defect in the enamel. As the cavity progresses into the dentin, it enlarges more and more quickly. Eventually the tooth has a small opening in the outer enamel and a great, hollowed-out area of dentin underneath it. Once enough dentin has been dissolved, only an enamel shell of the tooth is left. So one morning you're eating your toast and all of a sudden you feel a crunch. You've broken this outer shell of enamel and you can feel a big hole or cavity in one of your teeth. Contrary to what you might think, your tooth did not suddenly disintegrate while you were chewing your morning toast — your tooth has become the victim of all the previous activity of the S. mutans.

Do cavities cause pain?

In the initial stages of their formation, cavities may be quite painless. Depending where in the tooth they form and how far away from the nerve of the tooth they are, cavities and the cavity-forming process may remain unknown to you until the undermined "shell" of the tooth breaks. Even when that occurs, some people feel little discomfort. Others may feel sensitivity to sweets and cold as soon as the layer of enamel has been dissolved right through. Enamel is inert.

That is, it is a non-living substance that houses no nerves.

The underlying dentin consists of tiny microtubules that radiate from the nerve chamber outward toward the enamel layer. These tubules contain fluid. No sensation is felt as long as the ends of these microtubules are closed or sealed by enamel. However, once the enamel is dissolved, the outer ends of the tubules are open. The fluid inside is exposed to outside forces. Sweets and temperature changes cause fluid movement in the microtubules, which is felt at their other end (in the nerve chamber) by the sensing nerves. We perceive this movement as pain. However, each of us has a different pain threshold. So what one perceives as a minor sensation, another feels as major sensitivity or pain. The so-called pain threshold becomes pretty democratic once the cavity gets deep enough to reach the nerve of the tooth, and most people feel pain that they don't want to live with for long.

What happens if the cavity is not repaired?

Eventually the nerve of the tooth is affected by the enlarging cavity. As this happens, the blood vessels and tissues in the nerve chamber die off, leading to the formation of an **abscess**. I will discuss abscesses later in this chapter, in the section on root canal treatments.

The longer the cavity is allowed to progress, the more tooth material it destroys. Eventually, so much of the tooth may be dissolved that there is not enough of it left to repair by any means. When this happens, the remaining root must be removed and the tooth is lost. We will cover the consequences of such a loss in the section on prosthetic dentistry, also in this chapter.

Can cavities be reversed?

During the initial stage, when only the top layer of enamel has been dissolved, it is possible to stop a cavity from progressing further. At this stage, calcium from saliva can restore to a certain extent the calcium lost due to acid dissolution, if the shell of the tooth is still intact. Removal of the plaque and bacteria from the area right at the beginning of the stage may cause a reversal of the decay process. But it's impossible to reverse the destruction if the shell is already destroyed and a defect exists. No further decay will occur, however, if the area is kept clean from this point on. Why not? Because when the area is clean, no further acid will be present.

Unfortunately, this reversal happens very rarely. The reason is simple. A person can't feel tooth enamel being dissolved. Tooth enamel is inert, remember? So this cavity reversal would happen only if, purely by chance, that person started to thoroughly clean his or her teeth just as a cavity was starting to form.

How to prevent cavities

To prevent cavities you must remove — or at least control — their causes.

● You have to eat fewer sweets. With less sugar to work on, S. mutans have less to eat. So the bacteria don't multiply as readily and don't produce enough acids to dissolve your teeth.

● You have to keep your mouth meticulously clean. By cleaning your teeth with a brush and floss, you are removing plaque that harbors both bacteria and their sugary snacks. So you are reducing both causative factors. As well, you are reducing the time that the bacteria present in plaque are in contact with any one place on the tooth.

● You should consider fluorides. Fluorides greatly increase the resistance of enamel to acid. Fluorides bind chemically to enamel and provide a Teflon-like coating against bacterial acids.

If your drinking water is fluoridated, it will provide you with enough fluoride if you simply drink it from your tap at home. If you find that your drinking water is not fluoridated, you can take fluorides orally in tablet form (See chart in Chapter 3, page 53). Your dentist also can apply fluoride for you during your office visits, and he or she may recommend using fluoride rinses at home (see pages 52). Your dentist will help you decide whether your teeth are particularly susceptible to decay, and which form of fluoride you should use.

● You should have frequent checkups. Frequent checkups will allow your dentist to catch early on any cavities that are forming, before a lot of the tooth substance is destroyed.

How are cavities repaired?

Cavity repair is the most basic service that your dentist performs.

In most cases, unless the cavity is extremely small, the tooth must be anesthetized (frozen) first. This is done in various ways, which I describe in Chapter 2.

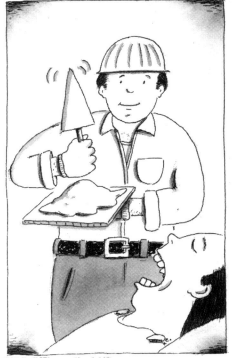

Once the tooth is anesthetized, the dentist uses an air-turbine handpiece to clean out any soft, partly-dissolved areas of the tooth. If only a small opening in the enamel is present, but a large cavity exists in the softer dentin underneath, the dentist sometimes has to enlarge the enamel opening to provide access for the cleaning. This is why people sometimes think that the dentist makes a big cavity out of a little one. Nothing could be further from the truth. The cavity was already large, but it was hidden under a shell of enamel. Without enlarging the opening, the dentist cannot remove the decayed (partly- dissolved) tooth material. Any weak and undermined areas of enamel are further removed once all of the decay, bacteria, and debris are cleaned out. The cavity is then shaped to receive and retain the filling material. When all of this is done, the inner walls of the cavity are lined with special cements and varnishes. These provide a layer of insulation between the filling material and the nerve of the tooth. As well, they seal the ends of the dentin microtubules that were originally sealed by the now-missing enamel.

At this stage, the filling material is placed into the cavity. It is shaped and contoured to replace the missing parts of the tooth and to restore the tooth to its original form.

Types of filling materials

Over the years, different materials have been used to restore teeth to their original form. Some — gold fillings, for example — have fallen out of favor due to cost. Others, such as porcelain inlays, are back in favor due to new bonding methods. However, the biggest question on everyone's lips today is whether or not the most commonly used type of filling — silver amalgam — is safe.

Silver amalgam fillings

Silver amalgam filling material has been around for nearly 150 years. Over the years, it has been improved a lot, and today's amalgam is very different from the original formula. However, its basic components — silver and mercury — are still at the heart of this filling material. Today's amalgam consists of microscopically fine spheres of silver and traces of other metals such as copper. Unlike the old times when the dentist mixed the silver and mercury with a mortar and pestle, the dentist today uses an amalgam which is precapsulated in a plastic container. Each capsule contains one dose of silver and trace metals in one compartment, and one dose of mercury liquid in another. The two compartments are separated by a thin foil partition. Just before use, the assistant squeezes the capsule, breaking the partition. The capsule is then placed into an amalgamator or mixing machine for thirty to forty-five seconds. After this, the capsule is opened and a soft metal filling is ready to be placed into a tooth. Because of the prepackaged capsule, the doses of silver and mercury are very precise. The free mercury is never touched and dangers of it spilling are greatly reduced. The silver amalgam is placed into a tooth cavity in small increments. Each increment is then compressed with a special instrument called a condenser. This ensures that the material flows into all corners of the cavity and that it is packed tightly and uniformly without any voids. After two to five minutes, the material hardens into a metal filling. During this setting stage, the material is shaped, using small carving instruments to resemble the portion of the original tooth it has replaced. Although it hardens in a few minutes, the filling has only a fraction of its final strength at this time. This is why a patient should not bite down on a new silver filling for a few hours after it has been placed. It takes about twenty-four hours for a filling to achieve its maximum strength.

Are silver fillings safe?
There has been a lot of controversy lately about the safety of silver fillings because of their mercury content. Amalgam fillings are approximately fifty percent mercury in content. The concerns include allergic reactions to mercury such as rashes or swelling in the mouth or neck area, long-term effects of mercury accumulation in the body such as neurological disturbances and, finally, environmental risks from mercury handling and disposal.

Over recent months, I have spent a considerable amount of time weighing the available evidence for and against the use of amalgam restorations in dentistry. I wish I could say that I have come to a definitive conclusion that I could state here. Unfortunately, not enough evidence exists at the moment to reach such a conclusion. The following is a brief outline of my findings, and of my current personal position.

Experiments performed in Canada on sheep and monkeys have shown that mercury from fillings collects in high concentrations in the kidneys and other organs of these animals. Furthermore, mercury in pregnant animals progressively concentrates in the placenta surrounding the fetus. Mercury also accumulates in the female animals' breastmilk, which would further contaminate the newborn animals.

Another study done in Sweden indicates that the amount of mercury released from fillings is about 1.7 µg (NOTE: µg = micrograms) per day.

The U.S. Food and Drug Administration (FDA) claims that 2 440 micrograms of mercury consumed per day is a safe limit. On the surface, this would suggest that we are well within tolerable levels. However, studies at the prestigious Karolinska Institute in Sweden suggest that mercury release varies with saliva type, oral hygiene, and diet. Other studies in Sweden show that mercury from amalgam fillings affects blood plasma level (the fluid part of the blood) whereas mercury ingested through eating fish affects mercury concentrations in the red blood cells. This would indicate that the two types of mercury are stored differently and thus the FDA figures may not apply.

Other Swedish studies have shown mercury levels in both urine and blood rising dramatically after all amalgam fillings are removed from human patients. However, within thirty days after the fillings are removed, the mercury levels *fall* even more dramatically — to twenty-five percent of the preremoval level it was in the urine, and to fifty percent of the preremoval level in the blood plasma.

Autopsies of people who have worked in dental offices show concentrations of mercury up to thirty-five times normal levels in some glands and organs.

If all these studies sound confusing to you, cheer up. You are not alone. Many international meetings have been held on this issue and the experts can't agree either. At one of these meetings, the assembled tall domes decided to come down firmly in the middle. They concluded that no clear evidence against amalgam exists, but that amalgam is toxicologically unsuitable as a dental filling material.

So if the experts can't agree, what do we do in the meantime?

I personally lean toward considering alternatives to amalgam fillings. It may be years before the jury is in with the final results, and in the meantime, better safe than sorry. Thanks to modern technology, we have an array of alternative filling materials to choose from. So I think that the prudent thing to do is to consider the alternatives in each situation as well as considering silver amalgam fillings.

At the risk of sounding as if I, too, am coming down firmly in the middle, let me add the following caveat: All of the alternatives to silver amalgam fillings are more expensive than amalgam. And there are a lot of other solid reasons why silver amalgam has been by far the most widely used type of filling material for more than a century. So before you decide what you should do, consider the following pros and cons.

What are the advantages of silver fillings over other types of fillings?

● **Strength**
Silver fillings are stronger than even the newest white filling materials.

● **Cost**
Silver fillings are still the least expensive form of restoration.

● **Ease of placement**
Silver fillings are much easier to place than the newer white fillings.

● **Durability**
Silver fillings wear better and last longer than white fillings.

What are the disadvantages of silver fillings?

● **Mercury content**
See discussion above.

● **Color**
Because of their color, silver fillings can only be used in posterior teeth.

● **Tensile strength**
Silver fillings are very strong when they are confined between walls of the tooth. However, when some of the walls of the tooth are missing, and the force on these fillings is directed so as to tear rather than to compress the fillings, silver amalgam is not the material of choice.

● **Lack of chemical bond to the tooth**
Since silver fillings do not bond chemically to teeth, they do nothing to help hold the remaining walls of the tooth together. And the junction between filling and tooth is not sealed as well as it is with a bonded white filling.

Bonded white fillings

What is bonding?

All white (or, more correctly, tooth-colored) fillings are bonded. Bonding is a term used to describe the mechanical and chemical attachment of the filling material to the tooth. The outer layer of a tooth — the enamel — is very smooth. Even under a microscope, the surface of enamel is extremely smooth. In order to attach a filling to this surface, the dentist must first roughen the surface to create in it millions of tiny microscopic dips, nooks, and crannies.

To roughen the enamel, the dentist applies an acid solution to it. This acid or etching solution has a jelly-like consistency. The dentist places the gel on the enamel around a cavity or in any area where something is to be attached to the tooth. Once the enamel surface has been etched (it takes thirty to forty-five seconds), it becomes microscopically rough. So if you looked at it with a microscope, you would see the millions of tiny dips, I mentioned above.

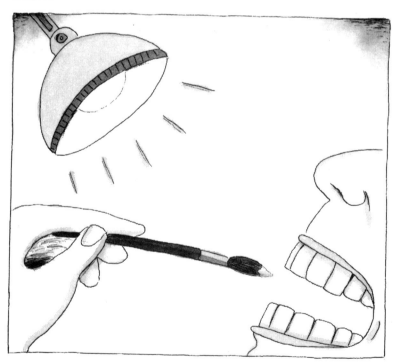

Then a thin coat of light-hardened bonding resin is painted onto the etched surface. The resin flows into and fills all the microscopic nooks and crannies. A strong light is shone onto the resin to cure or harden it. Once hardened, the resin forms a thin coat on the surface of the enamel. This coat of resin is held to the tooth by millions of finger-like projections made by the resin as it fills the irregularities in the tooth.

Now restorative materials can chemically bond to this resin surface and, indirectly, bond to the tooth. Until a few years ago the bonding procedure stopped here. Only the top layer of the filling was actually bonded to the top layer — the enamel — of the tooth. The part of the filling in the dentin underneath the enamel was not attached to the tooth. Recent research has helped develop solutions that can also condition dentin to chemically bond to filling materials. So far, this dentin bond is not very strong. But research is continuing with the aim of developing dentin-filling bonds that come close to the strength of enamel-filling bonds.

True bonded white fillings
A true bonded white filling is done in one sitting. The dentist places the filling material in the tooth cavity which was previously conditioned for bonding. The filling is then quickly hardened by exposure to a high-intensity light.

Until the 1980s, white filling materials were used only in front teeth because they weren't strong enough to withstand the much heavier biting force of the back teeth. The newer white materials are much stronger. Now many more back teeth are filled with white materials.

Advantages of true bonded white fillings

● **Esthetics**
The most obvious advantage of tooth-colored fillings is how they look. They can appear very natural because they come in a multitude of shades that can be matched very precisely to the color of the patient's teeth. They also can be used to brighten your present teeth (see the section on veneers, pages 97–100).

● **Little discomfort**
Because these materials bond to enamel and dentin, they reduce the need to cut retentive shapes into the tooth to keep the filling in place. So teeth can often be restored without any anesthesia, and with no pain or discomfort.

● **A better seal to the tooth**
Because bonding virtually fuses the surfaces together, it leaves no space between tooth and filling. So there is less potential for the recurrence of decay.

● **Preserving the tooth**
Because they bond to the tooth's walls, these materials help protect walls from further breaking and cracking.

Disadvantages of true bonded white fillings

● **High cost**
Because these materials require a lot more time and care to place, they are more expensive than conventional silver fillings.

● **Less durability**
White filling materials do not wear or last as long as silver ones. A silver filling has a life expectancy of five to seven years and many last much longer. The life expectancy of a white filling is two to four years. However, newer and better materials are being introduced all the time and some claim durability approaching or exceeding that of silver amalgam.

● **Less strength**
In small cavities these fillings seem to work well. However, in large restorations their strength is insufficient and inlays or onlays, or even full crowns, are necessary.

● **Difficulty of placement**
These materials are unforgiving of sloppy or inadequate application techniques. Dentists using them must be extremely careful. Not all dentists produce great results with them.

Gold or porcelain inlays and onlays

Inlays and onlays are used for larger restorations and require two appointments. At the first appointment, the dentist makes a mold of your tooth and cavity, which is sent to a dental laboratory. The lab custom-makes the gold or porcelain filling, which the dentist bonds into place on your tooth at the next appointment. These larger, lab-manufactured fillings are called inlays or onlays.

Inlays fit right into the cavity of a tooth. Onlays fill the cavity and also cover the outer walls of the remaining tooth, to protect them from fracturing. To simplify this discussion, I will combine the two and refer to all types as onlays.

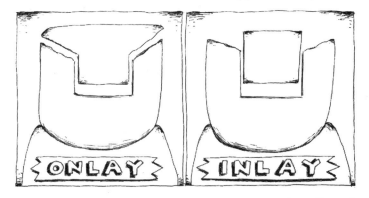

Here's how we restore your tooth with an onlay. First, the tooth is anesthetized, since any cavity requiring an onlay is a fairly extensive one. The decay is removed using a handpiece. The remaining tooth is shaped to receive the onlay. An impression or mold is taken of the tooth involved and of the surrounding teeth. A mold is also taken of the teeth in the opposing jaw. A wax (or other material) biting record is made to show how these opposing models mesh together in your mouth. The cavity is filled with a temporary filling until the next appointment. The laboratory makes an onlay out of porcelain or gold to fit into the model made from the impressions (molds). At your next appointment, the tooth is re-anesthetized, the temporary filling is removed, and the onlay is fitted and cemented or bonded into place. In the past, onlays were made exclusively from gold. With the advent of new, stronger porcelains and bonding techniques, tooth-colored porcelain onlays are now available.

Why an onlay instead of a regular filling?
Onlays are cast in the laboratory. Whether made of gold or
of porcelain, they have much greater strength than silver or
white fillings. This is true especially of shearing resistance.
Whenever the restorative material in a cavity is not completely surrounded by strong walls of the remaining tooth, it
is exposed to the shearing forces of the bite. A material is
needed here which will not break or crumble, and cast
materials are the only ones to date to meet this challenge.
In short, whenever a filling exceeds one third to one half of
the width of the biting surface of a tooth, that filling should
be an onlay or a crown.

Gold versus porcelain onlays
Whether you choose gold or porcelain onlays is a matter of
personal preference. Porcelain onlays are bonded to the
tooth, so they provide fewer opportunities for decay to form
between the tooth and the onlay. A well-made gold onlay
fits so tightly to the remaining tooth that it also leaves little
room for recurrent decay. Both seem to have about the
same durability and strength. However, gold onlays have
been used nearly ten times as long as bonded porcelain
ones. The final results are not yet in on porcelain onlays,
but from what we can see so far, they seem to wear well —
and they look great.

Why onlays cost more than conventional fillings
Onlays may cost three to four times what a comparable
filling does. They take more time, skill, and effort; plus
there are lab fees. However, we are comparing apples to
oranges here. You're asking for trouble if a tooth is destroyed to the point of needing an onlay, and you opt for a
filling. I see this in my own practice all the time. A patient
considers cost above all else and requests a filling. Then the
filling or remaining tooth breaks three or four times and
the patient realizes that an onlay would have lasted from the
start. Listen to your dentist. If an onlay is recommended, it's
for a good reason.

Crowns

Crowns, or as they are commonly called, caps, are a method of rebuilding the missing parts of the tooth and at the same time covering and protecting whatever still remains of the natural tooth.

What is a crown?

A crown is a metal or porcelain thimble that fits over the entire tooth and covers it all the way down to the gum line. The best way to think of a crown is as a protective shell around the tooth.

When do I need a crown?

You need a crown:

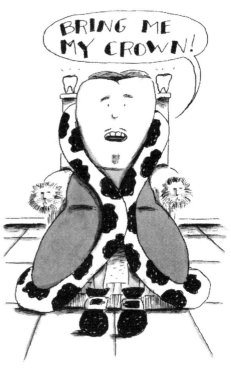

● when there is a very large filling in a tooth. If there are few — if any — walls surrounding the filling, or if these walls are very thin, you need a crown.

● when you have large, unsightly fillings and you want to make them look natural.

● if you have had a root canal performed on a tooth. *All* teeth that have had a root canal should have a crown placed on them.

● for cosmetic purposes. Crowns are one way to align and reshape front teeth. (See the next section on cosmetic dentistry.)

How is a tooth crowned?

First, the tooth to be crowned is anesthetized. Next, one half to two millimetres of tooth material is removed all around the tooth with a handpiece and a diamond bur (diamond drill). When they are told they will need a crown, my patients often say, "Oh, you're going to file my tooth down to a peg." They're wrong. Only one half millimetre is removed from some parts of the tooth. Sometimes nothing is removed at all. One to two millimetres are removed from other parts of the tooth to allow for the thickness of the porcelain crown. But in the end, there's still a very solid tooth left. It's just a little smaller. So don't think of it as having "pegs" under your crowns. Once the crown is on, that tooth is stronger than most filled but "unfiled" teeth.

Once the dentist has reduced the tooth the required amount, he or she places a medicated cord just under the gum, all around it, for a few minutes. When this cord is removed, its medication causes the gum around the tooth to shrink temporarily, exposing the border on the tooth where the future crown will end. Next, an impression (mold) is taken of the tooth and the adjacent teeth. As well, a mold of opposing teeth and a bite record are taken. These are sent to the laboratory, where the actual crown is made on plaster models made from the molds. The lab technicians have a model of the teeth which sit opposite from the crowned tooth, as well as a bite record of the teeth, so they can shape the crown to fit perfectly into the patient's present bite.

The tooth is protected by a temporary crown made of plastic or aluminum while the lab is making the crown. At the next appointment, the tooth is re-anesthetized, the temporary crown is removed, and the new one is cemented into place.

What keeps a crown in place?
When a tooth is shaped for a crown, its sides are made parallel to each other. The resultant shape is almost a cylinder. So the crown can only be dislodged straight up. In any other direction, it will bind onto the tooth, much as a drawer in an old-fashioned chest will bind if it's not opened along a perfectly straight line. To prevent the crown from dislodging upwards, the dentist places a special cement between the crown and the tooth.

How long will a crown last?
A crown is usually given a ten to twenty year lifespan.
However, I have many patients with crowns more than forty
years old. How long your crown will last depends on how
well you maintain your mouth. A crown will last many times
longer in a clean mouth than it will in one where plaque is
king.

How much does a crown cost compared to a filling?
A crown costs four to five times what a filling costs. But
when you consider how a crown protects your entire tooth
from future disintegration, along with the length of time it
will last, you can see that it is a good investment in the
health of your mouth.

What kinds of crowns are there?
There are three kinds of crowns.

● **All-metal crowns**
These are cast from precious metals such as gold, or from
non-precious alloys. Either type is excellent. The only
drawback to this type of crown is cosmetic — it is used in
back teeth only.

● **Porcelain bonded-to-metal (PBM) crowns**
These are metal crowns with a layer of porcelain on the
outside. The color of the porcelain is matched to the color
of the other teeth. Because the porcelain is bonded at all
points to the underlying metal, these crowns are just as
strong as the metal ones. Their advantage is that they look
like natural teeth.

● **All-porcelain crowns**
These crowns are made mostly for front teeth. The newer
porcelains are very strong and can be bonded to the underlying teeth. Their advantage is cosmetic. Because there is no
metal involved, the color of the underlying tooth can shine
through the crown, resulting in a much more natural
appearance.

Cosmetic dentistry

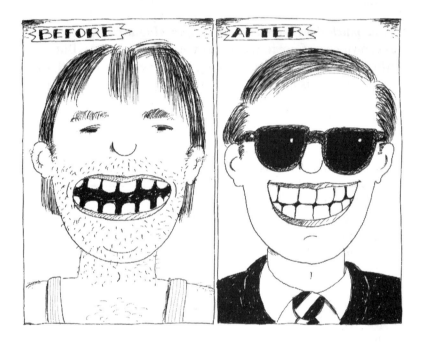

Cosmetic dentistry is a fairly recent branch of dentistry. Don't get me wrong, dentists have always tried to make their patients' smiles look as good as possible. In Hollywood, cosmetic dentistry has been around as long as the movies have. But until recently, improving your smile meant crowning all your front teeth. Only movie stars and their ilk took this expensive and rather bold step. The advent of bonding techniques and better resin materials has changed all that. Nowadays anyone can have a perfect, healthy smile with a lot less dental work involved.

To make it easier for you to understand just what can be done to improve your smile, I will list the possibilities, beginning with the simplest procedures and continuing to the most complex.

Cleaning and polishing your teeth

A young patient came into my office to inquire about bleaching his teeth. When I looked into his mouth, I couldn't believe my eyes. His front teeth were covered in *green* plaque. Here was an otherwise attractive young man, concerned about his appearance, who hadn't brushed his teeth in weeks! When I asked him why, he said his gums bled, so he tried not to disturb them! Of course, his gums bled *because* he didn't brush his teeth regularly. So the first thing you can do for a perfect smile is keep your teeth clean and your gums healthy.

A professional cleaning and polishing by your dentist will remove tartar buildup. It will also remove tea, coffee, or nicotine stains. If you are a heavy smoker, or if you drink a lot of coffee or tea, you may need to have your teeth polished every two or three months. If you leave the polishing for six months, you may spend four months with unsightly stains on your teeth.

If you have large white fillings in your front teeth, you will probably need more frequent cleanings and polishings because white fillings tend to be more porous than natural teeth. They retain more stains than natural teeth do, and they need to be repolished more often.

In short, the simplest way to a beautiful smile is to keep it clean.

Bleaching your teeth

A home bleaching kit may be just what you need to brighten your smile. Bleaching can produce spectacular results, especially in patients over forty whose teeth have yellowed with age.

First, your dentist takes a mold of your teeth. From this model, a plastic mouthguard appliance is made. This is a transparent plastic device which is closely adapted to your teeth. It is exactly the same as the mouthguard athletes use in such sports as hockey and football. (When you are not busy bleaching your teeth, you can use this appliance for protecting them during contact sports.) Usually we make mouthguards for the upper teeth only. But a mouthguard can be made for your lower teeth if they are prominent when you speak. You place two to four drops of bleaching solution into the mouthguard over each tooth to be bleached. Then you wear the mouthguard for three to four hours a day for seven to eight weeks. You should change the solution every one to two hours.

Bleaching is a very new method and no one knows how long the results will last. Periodic rebleaching may be necessary to maintain the effect. Some people who have used home-bleaching mouthguards have complained of slight tooth sensitivity and alteration in their bite, but they find that these problems seem to disappear once the active bleaching process is over. The cost of the mouthguard, solutions, and one or two office visits ranges from $150 to $250.

Recontouring or reshaping your teeth

Recontouring or reshaping teeth involves the careful and selective filing down of problem areas. It's a simple procedure and can produce surprising improvements. It is done without any anesthetic (freezing) and — believe it or not! — the patient doesn't feel a thing. This is because very little tooth substance is removed, and what is removed is taken from the non-sensitive outer layer of tooth, the enamel.

First, you and your dentist sit down with a mirror and go over areas that can be improved. You can do this in the dental chair holding a hand mirror, or you can use a model of your teeth. You'll be able to see the final result better on a model, especially if you want to make significant changes. But a mirror will be fine if you're just making minor adjustments. It is a good idea to watch in a mirror as the procedure is carried out. That way , if you think the result is not what you expected, you can ask your dentist to stop any time. Your dentist may have a lot of experience in cosmetic dentistry and a good idea of how the final result should look, but you're the one who will have to live with it. Beauty is in the eye of the beholder. Your opinion is the most important one here.

Common problems this procedure can correct include:

● A tooth on one side of your mouth longer than the other

A missing opposing tooth or a poor bite may cause a front tooth to overerupt. This means it will grow longer than the surrounding teeth or the corresponding tooth on the other side of your mouth. A simple way to correct this is to file down the excess length and to round off the edges to match the surrounding teeth. To ensure a permanent result, your dentist will have to correct the reason the extra lengthening occurred in the first place. The tooth may gradually lengthen again if the problem is not corrected.

● Pointy eye teeth

Some people have severely pointed upper or lower eye teeth which give a fang-like or Count Dracula appearance to an otherwise pleasing smile. It's simple to selectively file down and round off the points of such teeth and bring them into harmony with the remaining teeth.

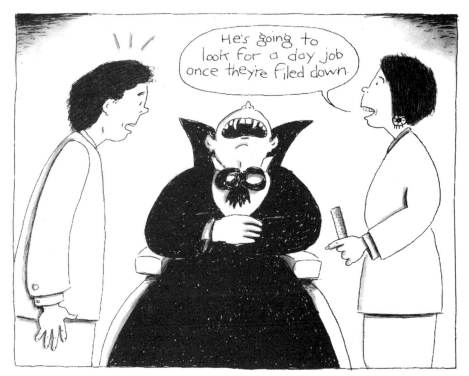

● **Chipped edges on front teeth**
Age or a minor accident may chip the front edges of a
tooth. Reshaping will even out the teeth to the deepest
portion of the chip. If the chips are very deep, they may
need to be filled in with bonded white fillings or veneers.
(See next section on white fillings.)

● **Teeth which look too masculine or too feminine**
I don't want to get myself into any kind of a sexist controversy here, but I think we all agree that some tooth arrangements are softer and more feminine, and some are more
robust and more masculine. Rounding off the far corners of
the front teeth achieves a softer look. Making the corners
more square and sharp achieves a more robust look.
Whether you think your smile is excessively masculine or
feminine is a highly personal matter and each case must be
evaluated individually. But if you suffer from either ten-
dency, you may need only simple reshaping to correct it.

Reshaping of teeth can greatly improve a smile. It is a fairly
inexpensive procedure. Most dentists' fees range between
fifty and two hundred dollars.

White fillings

Old, stained white fillings in the front of the mouth can be
unsightly. They should be replaced. There are many shades
of white filling materials now available, so there is no reason
to walk around with mismatched, discolored fillings. White
fillings can also be bonded to the outside of a tooth. They
can make short teeth look longer, small teeth look larger,
and skinny teeth look fatter.

Such white filling corrections are another pain-free
procedure. There is no need to anesthetize or freeze the
tooth, as the materials are painted on and bonded to the
outside of the tooth.

The dentist chooses a white filling material that perfectly
matches the shade of the tooth. The material is bonded to
the tooth and shaped with shaping burs and polishing discs.

This method works well for:

● **Fixing chipped or worn-out corners of front teeth**
White filling is added to make up the missing corner.

● **Filling spaces between teeth**
These spaces can be closed easily by bonding white filling
material to the adjacent teeth. If the space is very large, this
technique may not work because the resulting teeth will
look too wide. In such cases, crowning more teeth may be
necessary so that the extra width is distributed among four
or six teeth, rather than only two teeth. But white filling
material is the ideal solution if spaces are small.

● **Re-angling a tooth**
If a tooth is at a funny angle in the mouth, it can be made
to appear straight if white filling material is added to some
parts of it and not to others.

There are many other situations where this method works
well too. It is a relatively inexpensive way to correct your
cosmetic problems.

A word of caution: Durable as they may seem, white
fillings are still a hard plastic restoration. Plastic has its
limits, so you should avoid biting into hard foods with your
front teeth. As well, white fillings are the most likely to stain
with time. You may require more frequent cleaning and
polishing visits. In other words, you will now require more
care and maintenance. But that's a small price to pay for
looking and feeling great, don't you agree?

One-appointment veneers

"Veneering" means bonding a thin layer of a material onto
the visible parts of the tooth. This is done to hide stains and
discolorations, or to alter the color of the tooth. It may also
be done to alter the shape, position, or size of the tooth.

One-appointment veneering involves using the same
materials and technique as are used in white fillings. The
white filling material is bonded to the outside surface of the
tooth. But rather than merely fixing the chip or closing the
space between teeth, a thin layer of material covers the

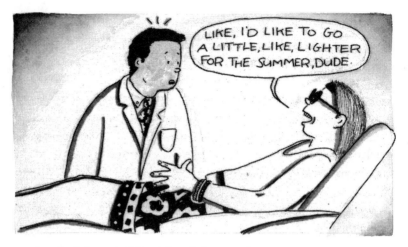

entire facial or visible side of the tooth.

This method is used if you want to lengthen or widen teeth or close spaces between them, and at the same time change the color of the entire tooth to match the adjacent teeth. It is also used if you want to change the color of all of your front teeth.

The advantages of this method of changing tooth color are:

● **No pain or discomfort**

● **Complete reversibility**
If you decide you don't like the result, the veneer can be removed and your tooth will be the same as before.

● **Lower cost than crowns or porcelain veneers**

● **Instant results from one appointment**

The disadvantages are:

● **Lack of strength**
As with all white fillings, you must avoid biting into hard foods.

● **More frequent polishing visits**
White plastic veneers stain more easily than porcelain veneers.

● **Reliance on the artistic talents of your dentist**
Let's be honest: some dentists are excellent clinicians but
are not artistically inclined.

Porcelain veneers

Porcelain veneers are also used to correct malpositioned
teeth or to cover unsightly ones.

As with other types of veneers, porcelain veneers can be
used to correct the color of a single tooth, or of all of the
front teeth. The difference here is in the material. Porcelain is much stronger than white filling materials. It does
not stain as easily. Porcelain also has a much more natural
appearance. It gives teeth a natural sheen that plastic filling
materials do not.

Porcelain veneers require two appointments. At the first
appointment, a mold is taken of your teeth and a shade or
color for the veneer is chosen. The molds are sent to a
dental laboratory where the actual veneers are made. A
week later, at the second appointment, your teeth are
cleaned and conditioned for the bonding procedure. The
veneers, which look like thin porcelain shells, are bonded to
the front or visible part of the teeth. The bonding is done
with visible light, which shines through the veneer. Both
appointments are discomfort-free. The final result is a set of
teeth that looks very natural.

Advantages of veneers:

● The results are beautiful and natural-looking.

● Teeth are as stain-resistant as natural teeth.

● They are durable. They last almost as long as crowns (ten
to fifteen years or more).

● They are completely reversible. If you don't like them,
you can have them removed and your teeth will be back to
normal.

Disadvantages of veneers:

● Two appointments are necessary.

● They cost almost as much as crowns.

● They do not strengthen weak or heavily-restored teeth.

To summarize: If your teeth need to be substantially brightened, or corrected in size, shape, or angulation, they will benefit most from porcelain veneers. They are my personal favorites because they provide lasting beauty with no treatment discomfort.

Crowns

All the ways discussed above to improve the shape and color of your teeth — cleanings, bleaching, white fillings, and porcelain veneers — are non-invasive procedures. This means they leave your teeth pretty well unchanged underneath the cosmetic treatment. In some situations, however, the change required is so extensive that none of these treatments will be sufficient. In these situations, crowning or capping is necessary.

Let's look at some examples where **crowns** are the solution.

● **Heavily restored teeth**
If your front teeth are so heavily restored that most of the natural tooth has been replaced by filling material, they will need crowns. A crown will cover and protect the remaining parts of the tooth and filling. It will hold everything together and will greatly strengthen your tooth.

● **Teeth that have been treated with root canals**
Teeth that have had root canal treatment often dramatically darken in color. Also, because there is no longer any blood circulation in them, they may become dry and brittle. This means they are in danger of breaking or splitting. Such teeth must be covered and strengthened with crowns.

● **Dramatically misaligned teeth**

"Buck teeth" — front teeth that project forward — are sometimes correctable with orthodontics, that is, straightening. This will take two or three years, however. Crowning them is a much faster correction. Crowns can correct this condition by realigning the teeth to their proper position.

● **A large space between the middle two front teeth**

This space can be closed by veneers, but the result would be two very wide teeth. A better solution, especially if you want to change the color of all of your front teeth, is to crown four to six of the front teeth. Each crown is made slightly wider than its underlying tooth. So if you have a space six millimetres wide, you can have six teeth, each one millimetre wider than normal, rather than having two teeth, each three millimetres wider. The final result looks tremendous.

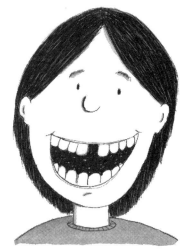

● **Missing front teeth**

A bridge — two or more crowns connected to a false tooth — is the ideal solution.

Crowns are usually done in two appointments. On the first, the teeth are anesthetized (frozen) and reduced (filed down) by one half to two millimetres all around. This is the part that concerns some people the most. "I don't want my teeth ground to little pegs" is the usual expression. But think about it for a moment. If your teeth are in a state where they need crowns, they will be many times stronger after they are crowned than they are now. The idea of "small pegs" is nonsense. The important thing is the final outcome. Will your teeth be better looking and stronger at the end of this procedure than before? The answer, if you require crowns, is an unequivocal YES.

Next, molds are taken of your teeth and sent to the lab where technicians make the actual crowns. In the meantime, temporary plastic crowns are made to cover the prepared teeth. These temporaries don't look nearly as great as your final crowns will, but they will see you through the week until your next appointment.

At the next appointment, your dentist puts your new crowns in place to evaluate them. Be sure that you have a mirror so you can approve them at this stage. It's too late for changes once they're permanently cemented in! It is a good idea to bring a friend or family member to this appointment to help you decide if the crowns suit you. Look closely at the color of the crowns. Natural sunlight is best for this evaluation — go outside if you have to. Size and shape are very important, too. Are the crowns too long or too short? Do they push out your lips or make them cave in? How do they look when you try a full smile? How do they look when you speak? Don't be afraid to ask your dentist for subtle changes. You will have to live with these crowns for many years. The crowns are cemented into place when you're fully satisfied with their appearance. Your new smile is *now* yours to keep!

Advantages of crowns:

● The color is stable. Porcelain crowns resist staining.

● They are strong. You can chew anything you would chew with your natural teeth.

● They are durable. They will last ten to fifteen years and often much longer.

Disadvantages of crowns:

● Two appointments are necessary.

● They are not reversible.

● The cost is high. Fees per tooth range from $550 to $650.

Crowns are a more involved form of treatment than white fillings or veneers. But crowns are the way to go if your teeth require strengthening or extensive restoration.

Orthodontics

Many cosmetic problems can be corrected by moving or repositioning teeth. This is called orthodontics. Some examples of situations that can be corrected with orthodontics are:

● **Widely-spaced teeth**
Widely-spaced teeth can be moved more closely together, orthodontically. As I write this book, I am into my third year of wearing orthodontic braces for this particular reason.

● **Crowded teeth**
Orthodontics can space them out.

● **Cross-bites**
When one or more lower teeth overlap upper ones, instead of the normal situation in which all of the upper teeth overlap the lower ones, the problem can be corrected with orthodontics.

● **Deep overbites**
The upper teeth completely cover the lower ones.

● **Misaligned teeth**
Teeth positioned at funny angles.

Many other situations can be corrected using orthodontics. Most of these involve wearing a full set of braces. The treatment may take six months to two or three years, and it will cost $1000 to $5000.

If you have healthy teeth and few restorations and you like the color of your teeth, then you would be a good candidate for orthodontics. You should still consider orthodontics if your teeth are healthy, even if your tooth color is a bit off (as my teeth are). You can always put porcelain veneers over your teeth once they are straight. That's what I plan to do. But if your teeth are going to require crowns to strengthen them, or if you don't want to wear braces for years, you shouldn't look at orthodontics as a solution.

Every person's situation is unique. Discuss your needs with your dentist. Perhaps your particular situation may require a combination of the above approaches. The main point I want to emphasize is that today everyone can have a gorgeous smile. Whatever it takes, if it makes you feel great, it will be worth it in the end.

Dentistry for children (Pedodontics)

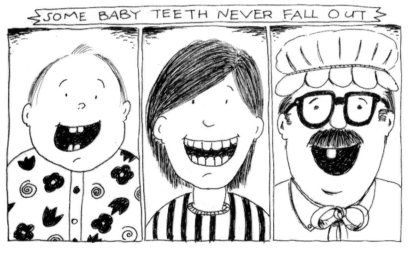

SOME BABY TEETH NEVER FALL OUT

The branch of dentistry that deals with the needs of children is called Pedodontics. In dentistry, we consider a patient to be a child until all the baby or primary teeth have fallen out and have been replaced by permanent teeth. This usually occurs between the ages of eleven and thirteen. Of course, there are exceptions to this definition. Some people are genetically missing some permanent teeth. Because of this, some of their baby teeth have never fallen out. Some patients in my practice still have a baby tooth at the age of fifty! And although I kid them about it, I don't really consider them to be children.

The goals of pedodontics are:

- to allow proper growth of teeth and jaws, including permanent teeth

- to allow proper chewing and speech functions

- to prevent any discomfort of dental origin

Let's analyse these three goals in detail and see how your dentist or pedodontist can help you achieve them.

Tooth development during pregnancy

One of the expectant mother's main concerns during pregnancy is proper nutrition. The mother-to-be should eat a proper balance of foods from the four basic food groups to ensure an adequate supply of nutrients and vitamins for the developing fetus. As far as the fetus' teeth are concerned, the two most important nutrients are calcium and vitamin D (to help absorb the calcium).

Calcium is found in milk and milk products such as yogurt and cheese. Calcium is vital for proper formation of bones and teeth, and vitamin D is necessary for proper absorption of calcium. Nowadays, vitamin D is added to milk at the processing stage.

It is also important for the expectant mother to ingest fluoride. Fluoride is absorbed by the fetus' forming teeth and is incorporated into the enamel of those teeth. It will act to make teeth more resistant to bacterial acids which produce cavities. Since only the baby teeth are forming in the unborn fetus, they will be the ones to benefit from fluoride during pregnancy. Unfortunately, at this time no studies exist showing optimum levels of fluoride supplements during pregnancy. The best source is fluoridated drinking water.

Teeth at birth

Most babies come into this world without any teeth. Every once in a while, a baby is born with one or two teeth already present. Although this may take its toll on the nursing mom during breast-feeding, being born with a tooth or two doesn't present any physiological problem.

As long as the baby's lips and jaws appear normal, the only concern with tooth development at this point is proper nutrition. Breastmilk will contain the calcium the baby needs. Vitamin D supplements are recommended for breast-fed babies. Fluoride supplements of 0.25 mg per day are recommended for babies six months to two years if the local water supplies contain less than 0.3 ppm of fluoride.

Two sets of teeth

We are given two sets of teeth during our lifetime. Although our jaws are quite small when we are children, we still need teeth for chewing our food. So during childhood we develop twenty small but efficient teeth. As we get older, our jaws get bigger. If we simply kept growing more teeth, we would end up with many small, weak teeth. Instead, nature replaces these small teeth with bigger and stronger ones as our jaws enlarge. Teeth are added, too, to give us a full complement of thirty-two teeth when we are fully grown.

First teeth

The timing and order in which teeth appear vary. The average times and order are shown on the next page.

A variation of six to twelve months from these times is not unusual. If your child varies from the average by more than that, you may want to talk to your dentist about it. The dentist may take X-rays to see if the teeth in question are present and, if so, what is holding them up.

TOOTH ERUPTION SCHEDULE

BABY TEETH

UPPER	WHEN TEETH APPEAR	WHEN TEETH ARE LOST
Central Incisors	8-12 months	6-8 years
Lateral Incisors	9-13 months	8-9 years
Canines (cuspids)	16-22 months	10-12 years
First Molars	13-19 months	10-11 years
Second Molars	25-35 months	10-12 years
LOWER		
Second Molars	22-30 months	10-12 years
First Molars	13-18 months	10-11 years
Canines (cuspids)	17-23 months	9-10 years
Lateral Incisors	7-16 months	7-8 years
Central Incisors	6-10 months	6-7 years

PERMANENT TEETH

UPPER	WHEN TEETH APPEAR
Central Incisors	7-8 years
Lateral Incisors	8-9 years
Canines (cuspids)	11-12 years
First Bicuspids	10-11 years
Second Bicuspids	10-12 years
First Molars	6-7 years
Second Molars	12-13 years
Third Molars (wisdom teeth)	17-21 years
LOWER	
Third Molars (wisdom teeth)	17-21 years
Second Molars	11-13 years
First Molars	6-7 years
Second Bicuspids	11-12 years
First Bicuspids	10-12 years
Canines (cuspids)	9-10 years
Lateral Incisors	7-8 years
Central Incisors	6-7 years

Teaching your child how to brush

As soon as there are any teeth, plaque starts to form on them. So your job as a parent is to teach your child how to keep that plaque off and keep those teeth clean.

I found the easiest way to introduce my own children to brushing was to give them a toothbrush and let them play with it. They would suck on it, look at it, crawl and walk around with it. It became their friend. You have to watch them, of course. A child falling with a toothbrush in his or her mouth can be seriously injured. You also don't want children cleaning the kitchen floor with their toothbrushes and then shoving them into their mouths. But with a little supervision kids can have a lot of fun with them.

You can teach your children how to brush properly and regularly once they are no longer afraid of a toothbrush. To do this, start by brushing their teeth yourself, twice a day, with toothpaste, or just with water if you find that they have a hard time spitting out the toothpaste. Make a game of it.

Make sure you brush all surfaces — the cheek side, the tongue side, and the chewing surface. My wife and I used to brush for our children first, then let them brush themselves. If you do it the other way around — let them brush first — you appear to be correcting them when it's your turn. If you let them brush after you, you let them feel that they are improving on your work. It makes them feel important. Ease up on supervision as they get older (around six or seven years of age). But do check up on them occasionally. We all know how easy it is to get into bad brushing habits.

When should your child start to floss?

Some authorities say you should begin using floss in a child's mouth as soon as there are two teeth next to each other. In theory, this is absolutely correct. Plaque from in-between teeth can only be removed with the use of floss. But in practice, it's a bit more difficult. Children have tiny mouths, and children wiggle a lot. They certainly don't have the manual dexterity to floss by themselves before the age of six or so. So you must floss for them. If you are gentle and get good cooperation, by all means do it as early as possible. But if it is a struggle and you end up cutting and hurting gums, give it up. You don't want to set up negative associations with daily oral hygiene. I would rather have the child start flossing later than have him or her learn to hate it early in life. Play it by ear until the child is five or six years of age. Introduce flossing as an integral part of toothbrushing after this age. That is, every night before going to bed.

Your child's first dental checkup

Unless you are aware of specific problems such as a discolored tooth, broken teeth, or visible cavities, you should leave the first dental visit until the child is about three years old. At this age, the child has enough reasoning ability to understand what is being done and why.

Usually, the first visit is an introductory one. In my office, it is spent showing the child around the office, giving the child rides up and down in the dental chair, and counting the child's teeth with a dental mirror and a counting probe. During this so-called counting, I get a pretty good idea of what, if any, problems there are. If we find no problems, we try to clean the child's teeth with a rotating brush and polishing paste. If this is too much for the first appointment, we don't push it. Usually we don't use fluoride treatment at the first appointment, as this may cause gagging and take away from the fun of the initial visit. The appointment ends with the child getting a new, small toothbrush and showing me the way to brush teeth. After the appointment, it's time for a sticker and a prize.

I find that if the first appointment is handled right, the next one six months later will be much easier. At this stage we usually get a chance to do a more thorough examination, take a couple of X-rays if any areas look questionable, and do a good cleaning and fluoride treatment.

When your child starts to lose baby teeth

Around six or seven years of age, when the child starts losing baby teeth, we must ensure that enough space is available for the next set of permanent teeth.

Dentists can estimate the size of the rest of the permanent teeth still to come once the four lower front permanent teeth have come in. They then can measure whether there is sufficient space in the jaw for all these permanent teeth. If permanent teeth appear too large for the size of the jaw, orthodontic intervention is necessary. Later in this chapter, in the section on children's orthodontics, I will talk in more detail about overcrowded teeth and shortages of space.

For now, we will consider situations that are normal. Parents are often concerned about the child's permanent teeth peeking through while the baby teeth are still around. This usually happens with the upper and lower front teeth. In the initial stages, this is not a problem. As the permanent teeth erupt further, they will usually push out the remaining baby teeth. Then the force of the tongue and lips will reposition the new tooth into its proper spot. In some cases, however, the newly formed permanent teeth are too far from the baby ones to effectively push them out. In these situations, it may be necessary to remove the baby teeth. I personally like to give these baby teeth a chance to come out on their own. I extract them only if there is no other alternative. Extracting teeth is not a pleasant experience for the child and, whenever possible, we should let Mother Nature do the job.

As we see the permanent teeth come into place, we are concerned with proper alignment of the jaws. There is an ideal position in which the upper and lower teeth should meet. We will discuss this at length later in this chapter, in the section on orthodontics.

What are the possible problems in the growing child's teeth?

Teething

As a baby's teeth are breaking through the gums, they cause the discomfort of teething. Most babies get grouchy and cranky as each tooth comes in, some more so than others. There really isn't much that can be done other than keeping the baby comfortable. We used a frozen, liquid-filled teething ring for our son and daughter. The cold contact eases some of the discomfort. Frozen juice cubes also help.

Rubbing the gums with your finger can help too. Some children find sucking on the bottle a relief; others find it painful. If sucking on a bottle seems painful for your child, offer a drink from a cup. It's important that liquids get in one way or another. On the positive side, remember that teething is not permanent. The discomfort lasts only a few days with any one tooth.

Baby bottle decay

A new baby can cause both parents a lot of stress, especially if the child is fussy and has difficulty falling asleep. Often, giving the baby a bottle is calming for the baby and induces sleep. This is fine as long as the bottle contains nothing but water. Sweetened juices, milk, or sweetened pacifiers that leave sugar on teeth throughout the night are an absolute no-no. They are a form of child neglect. This may sound rather harsh, but if you could see the ravages of decay caused when a baby falls asleep with a juice bottle, you would understand. Every once in a while I see a baby with front teeth rotten right down to the gumline from this practice. The child is in agony because the nerves on these teeth are exposed. And the worst part is that not much can be done for the child. Often there is not enough tooth left for a plastic crown (cap) or for a filling to be placed. Usually the teeth have to be extracted. For a two-year-old, this is severe trauma. It can leave memories about dentists that linger a lifetime.

The premature loss of teeth also leads to a loss of space for the future permanent teeth. It interferes with proper chewing and development of speech. Often lisps and other speech disorders result. These problems are very difficult to correct.

The simplest way to solve all this is to avoid it in the first place. *Never, ever* let your baby fall asleep sucking on a bottle unless the bottle contains only water.

Thumbsucking

Thumbsucking is a fairly common habit among young children. Often sucking on a bottle or pacifier provides the child with a sense of security. The child may resort to

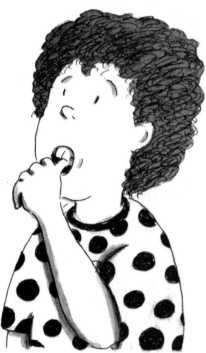

sucking on the next handy thing — his or her thumb — when these are taken away. Many authorities believe that prolonged thumbsucking is a result of emotional trauma. Often marital problems between the parents will trigger a thumbsucking habit or cause it to continue.

What are the consequences of thumbsucking?

They're unbelievable. Thumbsucking can force the upper front teeth to protrude outward (causing a Bucky the Beaver look), at the same time forcing the lower front teeth inward and causing crowding in the lower jaw. Over many years, thumbsucking literally changes the shape of the upper jaw and palate.

It's hard to believe that finger pressure alone can cause such changes but it does. The upper jaw becomes longer in the front and narrower in the back. When the teeth are brought together there is an opening between the upper and lower front teeth that precisely matches the size of a thumb.

What can be done to end a thumbsucking habit?

First, reason with the child. Thumbsucking should be
frowned upon and generally linked to negative parental
responses. Whenever the child is *not* engaging in the habit,
he or she should be praised and rewarded. This reinforces
the positive behavior the child is performing. This is the
carrot-and-stick method and it usually works well.

Some parents put mittens on their children at bedtime to
prevent them from gaining access to their thumbs. But
those children will probably try to remove the mittens and
then be punished for the secondary behavior of mitten
removal, rather than the primary one of thumbsucking.

Some dentists affix a "habit-breaking" appliance. This
usually consists of pointy wiring running along the roof of
the mouth. Whenever the child puts his thumb inside his
mouth, the wires interfere with the action. This often works,
but it would not be my first line of approach.

In my opinion, there is an underlying problem if the
carrot-and-stick approach does not work. I would suggest
spending time with the child to help sort out the underlying
cause for the behavior. A visit to a child psychologist might
help. Children, like adults, do certain things for certain
reasons. Learn what they are.

How can the results of thumbsucking be corrected?

Simply stopping the habit will allow the child's tongue and
lips to correct any minor existing damage providing the
child hasn't been a thumbsucker for long. If it's gone on for
a long time, the habit will cause more extensive damage
which will have to be corrected orthodontically. We will talk
about such corrections later in this chapter, in the section
on orthodontics.

Baby teeth that won't shed

The chart at the beginning of this section spelled out the
approximate times when baby teeth will be shed. As I said,
there is easily a six to twelve month variation within those
times. Your child should see a dentist every six months after
the age of three. Any abnormalities to this timetable can be
picked up during one of those visits. If a tooth is not being
shed on time there may be several causes.

● No permanent tooth

There may be no permanent tooth forming in the jawbone underneath the baby tooth. The pressure of an incoming permanent tooth is what makes a baby tooth fall out. This pressure causes the roots of the baby tooth to resorb (dissolve), thus facilitating its shedding. If there is no permanent tooth, the baby tooth will remain in place indefinitely. I have patients in my practice in their fifties who still have one or more baby teeth in their mouths. It keeps the child within them alive and well! Usually this means that the permanent teeth are genetically missing. Somewhere in the genes, there was never an instruction for the body to form this particular tooth. The most common teeth genetically overlooked are lower bicuspids (the teeth just in front of the large back molar teeth) and upper lateral incisors (the teeth next to the two central front teeth).

Nothing much can be done about this situation. All we can do is try to hold onto the baby teeth as long as possible and treat them as adult teeth.

● Damaged permanent tooth

The permanent tooth underneath may be damaged or facing in the wrong direction. This does not happen often. When it does, the situation must be evaluated by a dentist and an orthodontist. Sometimes it is possible to surgically attach a small hook to a misdirected tooth and bring it into proper position orthodontically.

● Baby tooth fused to the surrounding jawbone

A permanent tooth is present but for some reason — trauma for example — the baby tooth becomes fused to the surrounding jawbone. Dentists call this **ankylosis**. This fusion is strong enough to prevent the permanent tooth from pushing the baby tooth out. The baby tooth appears to be sinking among the other teeth as it remains in the same position relative to the jawbone, while the rest of the teeth continue to grow with the jawbone. The remedy for this is to extract the fused tooth as soon as possible. Although the permanent tooth is prevented from erupting in the face of the very strong fusion, it has no trouble coming into its proper position once the offending baby tooth is extracted .

Baby teeth that shed prematurely

Many parents have a lackadaisical attitude toward premature loss of baby teeth. They'll be lost eventually so why does it matter? they say.

Well, I'm here to tell you that it matters a lot. Firstly and most importantly, teeth drift. Whenever a tooth is missing, the surrounding teeth will drift or lean into the now-available space. When this happens, the permanent tooth that was under the lost baby tooth doesn't have enough room to come in. It will either come in on the cheek or tongue side of the other teeth, or it will come in only partly, or it will not come in at all.

Second, if front baby teeth are lost prematurely, speech patterns may not develop properly. Often children with this problem end up lisping, and mispronouncing certain sounds. These negative patterns may persist even when permanent teeth are in place. A lot of speech therapy may be necessary to unlearn these patterns.

Third, a baby tooth lost a year or two before its time, may cause the gum over the permanent tooth to become quite tough. This will make it more difficult for the permanent tooth to come in.

So every effort should be made to retain baby teeth until they are shed naturally.

Cavities in the baby teeth

Fluoridated water, improved nutrition and better awareness of the importance of regular tooth brushing have dramatically reduced the incidence of tooth decay in children. However, it still happens. It never ceases to amaze me how many parents don't see this as a problem. There is still a widespread attitude that decay in baby teeth is not important because these teeth will fall out anyway. In many provinces and states, neglect of children's teeth in this way is considered a form of child abuse, and I wholeheartedly agree.

Why repair baby tooth decay?

It's true that in time these teeth will fall out anyway. But until they do so naturally, there are many reasons for repairing decayed baby teeth:

● **Pain and discomfort**

Cavities in children's teeth cause children just as much pain and discomfort as do cavities in adults.

● **Danger to permanent teeth**

If a decaying baby tooth is left untreated it will abscess. The decay will penetrate deep enough to affect the inner nerve of the tooth, and cause infection and formation of pus. This endangers the child's general health, and often will cause damage to the forming permanent tooth in the jawbone directly underneath the baby tooth. The result may be a malformed permanent tooth susceptible to decay, or a severely discolored tooth.

● **Loss of space**

As a tooth decays, parts of it crumble away. This leaves a smaller tooth in place of the healthy normal tooth. This newly created space allows adjacent teeth to lean and drift closer together. So when the decayed baby tooth is eventually lost, either naturally or by extraction, it will leave insufficient space for the new permanent tooth. This leads to crowding, and to awkward positioning of teeth. A repaired baby tooth would have retained the proper space by preventing the neighboring teeth from drifting and tilting, and this problem would have been avoided.

How are baby teeth repaired?

Although baby or primary teeth are repaired much the same way as permanent teeth, their repair does involve some important differences.

● **Fillings**

If a cavity is small enough, it will require only a simple filling. Silver fillings are widely used on baby teeth. White fillings also may be used. However, white fillings don't bond as well to baby teeth as they do to adult teeth. In view of the controversy about mercury content in silver fillings (see pages 80–83), you the parent must make the decision about which fillings to use on your child's teeth.

● Root canals

In a baby tooth, the nerve is much closer to the outer surface (enamel) than it is in a permanent tooth. Because of this, decay gets to the nerve of the tooth that much faster, infecting it and causing an abscess to form. An abscess is a collection of pus at the root tips of the tooth. An abscess rarely causes the type of swelling in a child's jaw-bone that it would in an adult because a child's jawbone is thinner. Usually the abscess breaks through the bone next to the tooth and the pus drains in that direction. This is why you may notice a raspberry-like puffiness next to one of the baby teeth. This may even happen with a filled tooth, if the filling was very deep and close to the nerve. The pressure is relieved once the pus drains through the gum next to the tooth, and the child may no longer feel any pain. However, the danger of infection is still present, as is the danger of damage to the underlying permanent tooth.

To avoid these dangers, the dentist performs a baby version of a root canal. The dentist freezes the tooth, makes a small opening through the top or chewing surface of the tooth, and removes all the infected material from the nerve chamber and the nerve canals of the tooth. Unlike in a permanent tooth, little time is spent enlarging the nerve canals in the roots. Everything is cleaned and sealed with a medicated paste. A filling is then placed to fill the access opening.

It is very important to periodically recheck the area with X-rays to ensure that the infection has cleared up.

● Crowns

If a tooth is badly decayed to the point where it is severely weakened or no longer occupies as much space as it should, it is restored to its original form and size with a crown or cap. Crowns are invaluable aids to maintaining space lost due to decay.

Children's crowns, unlike adult crowns, are not custom-made to fit the particular tooth. The dentist has different-sized, prefabricated crowns. The closest in size is selected. The tooth is shaped and reduced about one millimetre all around. The crown is trimmed to fit over it and is then cemented into place.

Children's crowns come in two types — stainless steel for posterior teeth and plastic for front teeth. They usually last until the teeth are shed naturally, and are lost with them.

What if my child is already missing some teeth?

If, despite best efforts, a tooth is lost prematurely, an evaluation must be made to determine how soon the permanent tooth will come in. If the permanent tooth does not come in within two to three months, its space must be maintained and prevented from getting smaller.

The device used for this is called a **space maintainer**. Space maintainers come in different styles. If only one back tooth is missing, a metal band is cemented onto the adjacent tooth. To this band a hard wire loop is attached. The loop touches the tooth on the other side of the space, preventing the two teeth from coming closer together and closing the space.

If the problem involves missing teeth, it is corrected with a removable plastic denture-like appliance. The child is taught to wear this constantly. The denture can also replace any front teeth that are missing. In this way speech abnormalities are reduced.

What if some of the space is lost already?

If a tooth is lost prematurely and the surrounding teeth drift into the space, a **space-regaining appliance** may be necessary. This is an acrylic appliance that fits around all the other teeth in the jaw. Two spring-loaded wire arms extend into the space where the tooth is missing, one against each of the surrounding teeth. The tension in these wires is adjusted to push apart the teeth on either side of the space. The teeth are pushed back to their original position after the child has worn the appliance for a few months. Once that is accomplished, a band-and-loop type space maintainer is then made to hold the space until the permanent tooth comes into place.

Children in a dental office

If everything is okay when a child starts seeing a dentist (around the age of three), only regular checkups, cleanings, and fluoride treatments will be needed. These visits are easy and the child soon gets accustomed to them. To the dismay of their parents, children often look forward to dental visits!

What if work needs to be done?

In my experience, a child's response is greatly influenced by the parents' attitudes before and after each visit. Children model themselves on their parents, and if the parents are anxious about dental visits, children are usually terrified even before they step foot in the office. If you talk at home about how much *you* hate coming to the dentist, if you use words like drilling, pain, and needles, your child will absorb every syllable. If you talk about pulling teeth, hitting nerves, or climbing the ceiling before your dental visits, you shouldn't be surprised if you have to drag little Jimmy or Betty in for his or her visit.

Do's and Don'ts before and after a child's visit to the dentist

● If you can't say anything nice about your dentist in front of your children, don't say anything at all.

● **Don't** tell children not to be nervous or that "it won't hurt at all." It may never have occurred to them to be nervous, or that it might hurt. Your comments instill the idea.

● **Do** treat the upcoming appointment as casually as possible. If asked, talk about cleaning teeth, not about fixing them.

● Whatever you do, *never* use going to the dentist as a threat or punishment.

● It's fine to be sympathetic if you think your child has suffered. But try to be nonchalant after each appointment. Phrases like "oh, you poor thing," "well, now you're free for awhile," or "well, I am glad *that's* over with," don't do much to promote a child's cooperation on the next visit.

If I need to do work, I explain it to the child in positive terms during the appointment. It's amazing how well children behave during appointments if they don't come in with preconceived notions. If I see that a child is particularly nervous, I use laughing gas as a relaxant. We play games of jet pilots or astronauts to account for the "funny" mask that's worn. Usually, this is all it takes. Some dentists use premedication to control a difficult child. Drugs such as Valium are available in cherry-flavored syrups, and, taken by the child before the appointment, they work well.

If I can't reason with a child or I am unable to use laughing gas, I refer the child to a pedodontist, a specialist in children's dentistry.

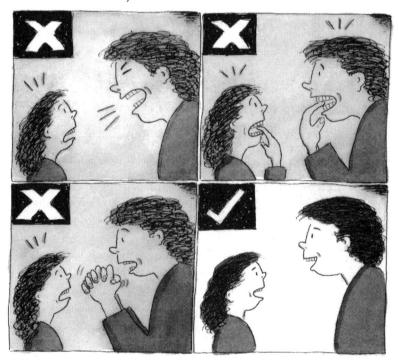

Pedodontists— dentists who only treat children

A pedodontist is a general dentist who has had one or more years of additional training specializing in children's care. Aside from having the extra training, pedodontists have the added experience of dealing with children all day long, every working day of their lives. Their offices are set up specifically for children. Many instruments and pieces of equipment are shaped like popular cartoon characters. Sometimes even the dentist and the staff are dressed up in cartoon-character costumes. Most offices are set up so that two or more dental chairs are together in one room. That way children can see each other during treatment and realize they are not alone. Pedodontists are more adept at premedicating children and are better able to handle a non-cooperative child. Often they are also associated with pediatric hospitals. Very difficult children in dire need of treatment can be handled in a children's hospital under general anesthesia. Fortunately, such situations are rare.

Moving and straightening teeth (orthodontics)

The textbook definition of orthodontics is this: Orthodontics is a specialty of dentistry concerned with the physical movement of teeth and jaws. Orthodontics is done for three reasons: to achieve a proper bite (a smooth fit between upper and lower teeth); to align (straighten) the teeth in each jaw; and to improve appearance.

So much for textbook talk. Most people think one thing when they hear the word orthodontics: beautiful, straight teeth. Good looks highlighted by a gorgeous smile. You get your teeth straightened to look better, don't you?

Yes and no. People want to look their best, and straight, even teeth are a big step toward that goal. A great smile is a tremendous psychological boost to anyone, regardless of age. Everyone knows how cruel children can be to their peers in the schoolyard, and a kid with buck teeth is an easy target. Adults persecute one another more subtly but the effects can be just as destructive. Crooked, unsightly teeth are a social handicap that can jeopardize everything from job prospects to success in love.

But there are other reasons for orthodontic work besides cosmetic ones. Properly aligned teeth and a good bite are vitally important to the health of your teeth, gums, and jaws. A poor bite can stress teeth beyond their limits and cause them to loosen, chip, or wear prematurely. It can even lead to abscesses.

Improper bites also stress the jaw joints and can contribute to painful and limiting conditions such as TMJ Syndrome, which I discuss later in this chapter. And the difficulty of cleaning around misaligned teeth can lead to periodontal (gum) disease.

Can my regular dentist do orthodontic work?

Most dentists are taught to perform orthodontic treatments during their basic training. But if a dentist wants to hang out a shingle as an orthodontist, he or she has to specialize, which means an extra two to three years of training in orthodontics.

This doesn't mean you have to go to an orthodontist if you need orthodontic work. Some general practitioners take a personal interest in orthodontics, and have a particular affinity for it. They may take extra courses and seminars in the field to improve their skills. More training and experience allow them to treat more complex cases.

But in general, you will find that your regular dentist will treat only simple tooth alignments and cross-bites. He'll refer more intricate problems to an orthodontist.

If you or your child have what you feel to be a complex case — for example, skeletal problems involving the size and position of the jaw — you may want a second opinion if your dentist wants to treat it independently. Honesty and openness are the keys to success in situations like this. Tell your dentist about your doubts. He or she should be willing to provide you with the names of two or more specialists. You might also ask for names of previous patients of your dentist who have had similar treatments. Your dentist may be happy to arrange for you to talk to these patients or their parents.

A cautionary word about getting a second opinion: Be sure you're comparing apples to apples. That is, be sure both dentists are offering you the same types of treatments. Specialists are likely to suggest complete, ideal treatments to correct all the problems. Your family dentist may have been trying to correct only a cross-bite or some other simple problem. You may or may not want a complete treatment. One way to be sure of what you are discussing is to ask all dentists involved to list in writing what they plan to do.

Children's Orthodontics

One of the major decisions you must make as a parent is whether or not your child should have orthodontic treatment. It's a big decision for several reasons. First, there's the cost. Many a divorce agreement has foundered over who is responsible for paying the orthodontist! Full-scale orthodontic work **is** a major expense that will run up to several thousand dollars. Before you sign on the dotted line, you want to be sure it's going to be worth it.

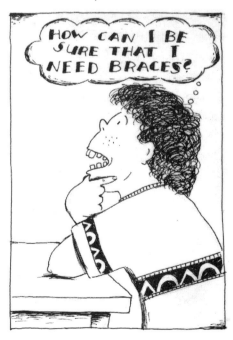

Your next question may be something like, "How do I know I should agree to fix Johnny's bite? He's only seven years old and he looks fine to me. How can I be sure the dentist is right and that Johnny is developing a severe overbite, or that his jaw will be too small for his permanent teeth?"

And last but certainly not least, you must ask yourself if you and your child are willing to make the enormous commitment of time, effort, and cooperation that orthodontic work requires over not one year, but over a number of years.

Don't be intimidated.

Let's start with your child's diagnosis. We dentists are notorious for using complicated language. Don't be intimidated if your dentist describes your child's orthodontic problems, and the kinds of treatments you might consider, in confusing technical terms. Your child's problems probably fall into one of three broad areas.

The three most common orthodontic problems of children

Jaw size versus tooth size

Too many teeth for the jaw

Sometimes nature seems to underestimate or overestimate how large the jaws need to be to contain all of the teeth. Even if you don't have any extra teeth you may have teeth too large to fit into your jaw. The result is crowded, bunched-up teeth.

The treatment: Create more room by extracting teeth. Usually the teeth extracted are the bicuspids. These are the small back teeth just in front of the big molars at the back. Usually one is extracted on each side. A total of four teeth may be extracted if both top and bottom jaws are crowded.

Deciding to extract teeth is always a tough decision for parents to make. Dentists are supposed to save teeth, not pull them, aren't they? Yes, that's true, but I suggest you try looking at the benefits. Is it not better to sacrifice four teeth so that all the others can remain healthy and well-aligned? Believe me, dentists and orthodontists think long and hard before reaching a decision like this. We make such a decision only when the benefits far outweigh the losses. Once the permanent teeth are removed, the remaining teeth are moved into alignment in the spaces opened up. This is usually done using braces, and takes two to three years.

Sometimes, if we discover early on that the child's jaws will not be able to accommodate all the teeth, we perform **serial extractions**. We extract the baby teeth in a certain order, at certain stages of growth, which allows the permanent teeth to come in straight. Eventually the last incoming permanent teeth are extracted, leaving all the teeth in front of them in proper alignment. This type of interceptive treatment minimizes the amount of orthodontics required later on.

Too few teeth for the jaw

Sometimes the opposite problem exists. That is, the jaws are larger than the sum total of the teeth. This means that spaces exist between the teeth. If no other bite problems exist, this problem is purely cosmetic. The teeth can be brought together with braces or, in mild cases, with a removable appliance. The treatment takes one and a half to three years. The biggest problem is long-term maintenance of these teeth in their new positions. They tend to spring back and spaces or gaps reopen because there is nothing to hold the teeth back. The only solution may be to wear a retainer at night, indefinitely.

Skeletal problems

Skeletal problems are those with the jawbones rather than with the teeth themselves. The upper jaw may grow more, and faster, than the lower jaw. This leads to protruding upper teeth or a "Bucky the Beaver" look.

Conversely, the lower jaw may grow too much, which leads to a hag-like protruding chin and a caved-in mid-section of the face.

Skeletal problems also occur side-to-side and result in one jaw being severely narrower than the other. This prevents a healthy bite between upper and lower teeth.

The treatment: Skeletal problems are best treated during a maximum growth period. The pre-pubescent growth spurt occurs around ten to twelve years of age for girls and eleven to thirteen for boys. During this growth spurt, it is possible to hold back one of the jaws, allowing the other one to catch up.

If the upper jaw is growing ahead of the lower one, it is held in place with a **headgear** while the lower one catches up. A headgear is a heavy wire arch that attaches to the upper back teeth. The outer arms of the arch come out of the mouth and encircle the face ending just in front of each ear. An elastic band is attached to each end, and in turn attaches to a neck strap or a small skullcap. The idea is to use the neck or the back of the head for anchorage to pull the upper jaw backwards.

To say that headgears are not very popular with parents or children is a vast understatement. They are **not** pretty. Unfortunately, no one has thought of a way to disguise them or to make them more acceptable for a child or teenager to wear. Unlike many retainers, they must be worn at least twelve to sixteen hours a day. Usually the child wears the headgear at home after school, as well as through the night while sleeping. Headgears must not be worn during any sports activities. This includes bicycling; playing on swings, slides or other equipment in a playground; or any other activity where the child might fall. Horsing around at home is forbidden for the same reason: The child can get badly hurt if pushed or jostled while wearing a headgear.

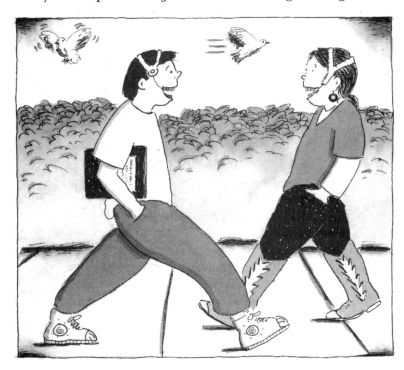

If headgear treatment coincides well with the pre-pubescent growth spurt, it accomplishes what it is supposed to do reasonably quickly — within twelve to twenty-four months.

Weary parents will attest to the fact that a great deal of supervision is required to encourage proper wear of headgear. Because of this resistance to headgear therapy, many dentists and orthodontists are using other methods such as **bionators**. These are large removable appliances worn inside the mouth. They work by pitting the upper jaw against the lower one, especially during functions such as swallowing. Again, these appliances only work if they are worn regularly. So proper compliance is a must. Many dentists and orthodontists will insist on parents keeping a daily log of how many hours the appliance is actually being worn.

Bite problems

Even when a child has jawbones that are well aligned and teeth that are not crowded, he or she may have upper and lower teeth that do not bite (mesh) properly.

Normally, upper teeth rest on the outside of the lower teeth, overlapping them. One or more upper teeth sitting on the inside of the lower ones, is known as a **cross-bite**. Cross-bites put tremendous strain on the teeth involved. Fortunately, they can be corrected easily within six to nine months, with a removable appliance.

A more severe bite problem is the **open bite**. In an open bite, the back teeth bite normally but the front teeth do not come together. Open bites are usually the result of habits such as thumbsucking (see pages112–113). Most children suck their thumbs as a result of emotional trauma. Finding the source of this trauma is the key to breaking this habit. Once the child is willing to cooperate, he or she has a small appliance made to fit inside the mouth. This appliance will get in the way whenever the thumb is put in the mouth, and be a "reminder" to stop. If children stop thumbsucking early, their open bites can be corrected quickly with a removable appliance. Often, however, the habit goes on into the early teens. By then, not only are the teeth moved by the thumb; often the shape of the upper jaw is changed, too. It becomes elongated at the front and narrowed at the back. This requires extensive treatment lasting two to four years.

When should my child begin orthodontic treatment?

The time to see an orthodontist is fairly early. Usually the best time for a first consultation is at age seven. If there is an orthodontic problem, it is possible that treatment at this age will reduce the amount of treatment required later on. Serial extractions, for example, should be started at this time.

If your dentist believes that early intervention will not yield any results, it may be necessary to wait until the child is ten before treatment can begin. Children go through a big growth spurt between the ages of ten and thirteen. Catching and using this growth to aid treatment allows your dentist to alter dramatically the total time of treatment and the final outcome. Your dentist and orthodontist can predict quite accurately when your child's growth spurt will occur by doing a close analysis of two things: his dental records and special X-rays of one of your child's wrists.

Strange as it may sound, a special X-ray of the child's hand shows the development of a unique bone. This bone provides the best estimate of the bone development stage of your child. This knowledge is critical to proper timing of the treatment of skeletal problems.

Diagnosing your child's orthodontic problems

The most crucial part of any orthodontic treatment is the initial diagnosis of the problems and their locations. To make a proper and complete diagnosis, the dentist must:

● **Measure the size of the child's jaw, and of each individual tooth.**
X-rays and models of the teeth are used to do this.

● **Carefully assess the child's facial features.**
The dentist must consider any asymmetries such as a nose or a chin displacement to one side or the other, defects such as protruding lips or nose, or a protruding or receding chin.

Much more than your child's teeth and jaws are at stake here. You and your dentist must be aware of your child's face as a whole. For example, treatment which calls for moving top teeth back may accentuate an already prominent nose. What will this nose look like when the orthodontic treatment is completed? Will you then have to consider a surgical nose reduction? If you're not prepared to do that, you may have to decide whether your child would be better off with protruding teeth or with a protruding nose.

● **Analyse the child's bite.**
The dentist must assess how treatment will improve the way the upper and lower teeth fit together.

● **Take complete X-rays.**
Special X-rays of the skull in profile, called **cephalometric X-rays**, must be made and analysed before any orthodontic treatment. These specialized X-rays give angle measurements between the skull, the jaws, and the teeth (however they are positioned). They also uncover any skeletal problems.

Ordinary X-rays must be taken too. They may show abnormalities such as missing permanent teeth, or extra teeth that will interfere with proper eruption and alignment.

And, as I explained above, an X-ray of the child's wrist may be required in order to best estimate the stage of bone development your child is in.

● **Perform a full dental checkup.**
This will be done by your family dentist. Orthodontic work cannot begin until all regular dental work is completed. There is little point in straightening decayed or broken-down teeth. And it is much more difficult to perform restorative work once braces and other orthodontic appliances are placed on teeth.

● **Assess the child's oral hygiene.**
If they are not up to par, proper oral hygiene habits must be developed before treatment begins. Keeping a clean mouth is both more important and more difficult for the child once braces or other appliances are in place. Your

orthodontist should stress how important it is to keep the mouth and teeth flawlessly clean during orthodontic treatment.

● **Talk to you and your child fully and frankly about the entire orthodontic treatment.**

It is important for everyone to understand the commitment and cooperation orthodontic work requires. It's a commitment that lasts years, and it should not be entered into without careful thought. You will have to supervise closely your child's daily oral hygiene and wearing of appliances, and your child will have to be prepared to cooperate, too. Orthodontic treatment requires a large commitment from parent *and* child. Make sure you are both ready for it.

After following the above steps, the dentist or orthodontist makes a diagnosis and draws up a treatment plan. If, at this point, you decide you want a second opinion, you can request that all X-rays and models be sent to the other dentist or specialist. This will substantially reduce the cost and trouble of seeking a second opinion. As well, the child will not be exposed to unnecessary extra X-rays.

Braces

They're not what they used to be.

Braces are used to align and straighten crooked teeth, to close up spaces, and to correct poor bites. Most orthodontic treatments require braces. Only very simple problems can be corrected without them.

Until the advent of bonding, all braces were made of metal attached to the tooth by a metal band. Now braces are bonded directly to the tooth. You can get braces that are metal, clear plastic, or porcelain. Metal braces are the least expensive but the most visible. Clear plastic ones are more expensive but less visible. Some orthodontists don't like using plastic braces because they are not as sturdy as metal braces. Porcelain braces are the most expensive and the sturdiest. And they are almost invisible.I have been wearing porcelain braces for the past two years and people who see me every day are barely aware of them. The wires, which fit into the brace on each tooth and do the actual moving, however, are still metal. The elastics that hold them in place are usually clear and invisible. But lately, brightly-colored wires and elastics are all the rage. Every cool teen is wearing neon pink and blue wires and elastics this season.

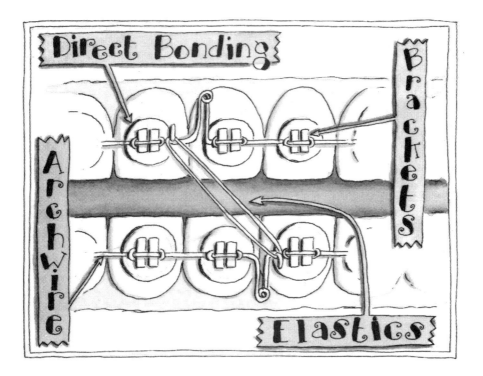

Do braces hurt?

As the orthodontist puts on the braces, there is no pain. Once all the wires have been connected onto the braces, they will cause the child to feel pressure on the teeth. This will last a few days after the initial appointment and after each monthly adjustment appointment. Some orthodontists suggest using over-the-counter pain relievers to alleviate this discomfort. Others provide a plastic wafer which relieves discomfort when your child chews on it vigorously.

How long must braces be worn?

Braces usually are put on between the ages of ten and
thirteen and are worn for eighteen to thirty-six months.
They are fixed to the teeth, and the child has to put up with
them whether he likes it or not. In some cases, the orthodontist may prescribe elastics worn between top and
bottom teeth. It is crucial that these be worn constantly and
that they are changed daily.

Eating with braces

There are some limitations on what the child can eat when
wearing braces. For the first few days after each adjustment
visit, the teeth may feel quite tender. During this time, the
child may be comfortable eating soft foods only.

Throughout treatment, the child wearing braces should
avoid crunchy foods such as nuts and popcorn. The same
goes for sticky foods like toffee. Foods like this can cause
the braces to pop off or the wires to bend. Fruits such as
apples and pears should be cut up before they are eaten
and should not be bitten into with the front teeth. All other
normal foods are fair game.

Cleaning around braces

Anyone who has worn braces knows how important it is to
work extra hard at cleaning the teeth. All the hardware adds
dozens of additional nooks and crannies where plaque can
collect. So it is important to take extra care to make sure
your child's oral hygiene is topnotch. With braces, there are
three zones to clean on each tooth: above the brace, below
the brace, and the brace itself. A small-head children's
toothbrush can best negotiate these small surfaces.

Flossing is complicated by braces, too. The best way to
floss around braces is to thread the floss in-between the
teeth with a plastic floss threader.

Small interproximal brushes can also be used to get in-
between teeth.

A water irrigator is a great way to flush food and debris
from in-between braces. I suggest a weekly fluoride rinse to

help prevent decay in hard-to-reach places.

And finally, don't forget your child's regular dental checkups. Most orthodontists don't check teeth for decay during orthodontic treatment. This is your regular dentist's job. The added difficulty of keeping teeth clean when wearing braces means regular checkups are extra important. What's the use of having straight, rotten teeth?

Retainers

Teeth try to spring back to their former positions once braces are taken off. A retainer must be worn full-time, day and night, for six to twelve months after the braces come off. After that, nightly wear for the next six to twelve months is usually enough to keep the teeth from relapsing. The exact length of time a retainer must be worn varies with the severity of the original condition.

Fees

Fees for orthodontic treatment vary greatly. Simple procedures such as cross-bite corrections requiring removable appliances cost between $400 and $700. Usually there is an up-front fee for the appliance, plus a fee for each adjustment appointment.

Full braces may cost $3000 to $5000 for the complete treatment. This includes an up-front fee of $500 to $1500, with the remainder paid off monthly over the course of the treatment.

About sixty percent of insurance plans cover orthodontic treatments. Usually they have a lifetime maximum of $1000 to $1500 and limit treatment to children under the age of sixteen.

It is best to have your dentist or orthodontist send an estimate to the insurance company ahead of time. Then you will know in writing how much of the fee will be reimbursed to you.

Having a written estimate is also a good idea, in case any disagreements arise during the course of the treatment.

Adult orthodontics

It's never too late.

Until a few years ago, orthodontic treatment was considered
something for children only. Today, adult orthodontics is
one of the fastest growing segments of dental care. I myself,
at a tender age of thirty-something, am just finishing my
orthodontic treatment. I have a patient who began her
orthodontic treatment at fifty-seven and got to enjoy beautiful straight teeth on her sixtieth birthday. You are never too
old to straighten your teeth.

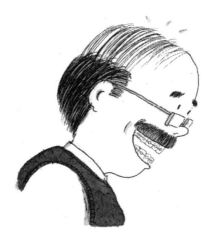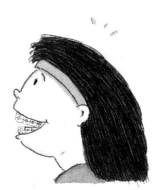

Types of correction

The types of orthodontic work done on adult patients range
from very minor tooth uprighting to major, surgically-aided
skeletal corrections. Let's discuss some of these, starting
with the simplest ones.

Tooth uprighting

Wherever one or more teeth are lost, they leave a space into
which the adjacent teeth move and tilt. This creates spaces,
in-between neighboring teeth, which can be unsightly and
which can create areas where food and plaque can accumulate. The tilted teeth also present uneven tilted surfaces that
interfere with proper bite. An untreated improper bite, left
long enough, creates problems for the jaw joints. The

solution is to replace the missing teeth with a bridge or a partial denture. However, it is often advantageous to up-right the existing teeth and to bring them closer together before tooth replacement.

Enter orthodontic treatment. Braces are usually placed only on the involved teeth. Springs and elastics are used to upright and align tilted and drifted teeth. This process may take six to nine months. It is painless and easily accomplished. None of your friends will even notice, if the teeth involved are in the back of the mouth. A bridge or partial denture is made once the teeth are repositioned. The bridge will hold the teeth in their new places without the need for any other retainers.

Minor cross-bites

If a single front tooth is biting in reverse to all the others, it creates a condition called a **cross-bite**. It can be easily corrected with a removable appliance that has a spring which pushes the offending tooth back into line with its neighbors. Treatment time is three to six months. The onus is on you to wear the appliance as much as possible. You should wear it twenty-four hours per day, including when you eat and sleep. The appliance is removed when you clean and brush your teeth in the mornings, at night, and after every meal or snack. However, if you have one or two big social events during treatment, you have the comfort of knowing that you can take the appliance off for those few hours.

The force of the bite will keep the tooth in its proper place after the cross-bite is corrected, negating the need for retainers.

Crowded teeth

Crowding often results if your teeth are too large to fit inside the space provided by your jaws. Crowded teeth are more difficult to clean and often develop decay faster than straight teeth. As well, the gums around crowded teeth are often forced into funny positions that aren't stable. The result is increased risk of gum recession and periodontal disease and, of course, a smile that leaves something to be desired.

Selective **discing** or grinding may open up the necessary

space if the crowding is mild. Approximately one-half millimetre is filed off the sides of each front tooth. This is painless, and the part of the tooth filed won't be missed. The result is one-half millimetre times two sides times six teeth — or six millimetres of extra space. A removable appliance worn for nine to twelve months after the filing will create a perfect, healthy smile.

Sometimes, however, six millimetres is not enough to align all teeth, and one back tooth on either side must be extracted. Substantial tooth movement is required, so braces are necessary to align all teeth and properly close all remaining spaces. This is an eighteen to twenty-four month treatment.

You will have to wear a retainer, once your teeth are in their proper places, for an additional six months full-time, and then six to twelve months at night only.

Skeletal corrections

An upper or lower jaw grossly out of alignment is a skeletal, and not a tooth-related problem. This means that the upper or lower jawbone is too far forward or too far back to properly meet with the other. The net result is that the chin is either very pronounced and juts forward, or it is greatly receded, and makes the face look chinless.

In a growing child, the problem is corrected by altering the growth of one or the other jaw. In adults, because growth has stopped, surgical correction is necessary. An oral surgeon working in conjunction with an orthodontist can correct the jaw position. After surgery, upper and lower jaws are tied together with braces until healing is complete. This takes three to six months, during which the jaw heals. While the jaw is healing, only liquids can be taken through a straw. So a side benefit may be a loss of weight. Think about it — after a few months, you get a new face and a new figure. What a deal!

After the jaws are healed, they are untied, and the braces on upper and lower teeth accomplish any final bite corrections. The end result is a dramatic improvement in appearance, as well as a proper bite relationship. Several patients in my practice have undergone this procedure and are very happy with the results.

Who does orthodontic treatments?

Most dentists know their limits. Simple uprighting or alignment can usually be handled by your regular dentist. But an orthodontist or an oral surgeon should perform the treatment when teeth are extracted to create more room, or when surgery is required.

Orthodontic treatment is included in most dentists' basic training. Although full braces are usually done by an orthodontist (who has undergone two to three extra years' training as a specialist), they may be done by some general practitioners as well. If your dentist wants to tackle this, you may want to see some previous cases first. Your dentist should be happy to refer you to patients he or she has treated before.

Are there any reasons I should not consider orthodontic treatment?

One of the few dental reasons not to consider orthodontic treatment is the presence of periodontal disease. Any gum disease inside your mouth must be treated before orthodontic treatment begins.

Weak teeth with heavily receded gums don't do well with the added pressure of orthodontic appliances either. If you're in doubt about the well-being of your gums, you may want to consult a periodontist before proceeding with orthodontic work.

Braces

Braces are not what they used to be. There are now several types to choose from, none of them unsightly. The most popular braces among adults are **porcelain braces**. Porcelain braces are very unobtrusive, cosmetically. They are bonded to the teeth, and clear elastics are used to keep the aligning wires in place. I have been wearing porcelain braces for the past two-and-a-half years, and I know that very few of my patients have even noticed them on me.

Invisible braces are also popular with adults. These braces are bonded onto the tongue side of each tooth so that they can't be seen from the front. Not all cases can be corrected using these, but they're worth asking about.

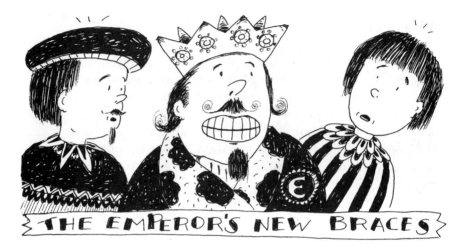

Are braces painful to wear?

No. Their placement is painless. You do feel some pressure when they're first put on, and after each adjustment appointment. Soft foods are ideal for those times. Otherwise you feel no discomfort. Some people find that braces irritate their tongue and cheeks. Orthodontic wax can be used to reduce this. You just place a piece of the wax over the offending braces to allow your cheeks or tongue a chance to heal.

Costs

Costs for orthodontic treatment vary depending on how complex it is. Simple uprighting of one or two teeth may cost $200 to $400. Full braces run $3500 to $5000 for the entire treatment. Surgical procedures are usually done in the hospital and may be covered by your medical plan.

Don't forget that treatment may take up to three years. You can space your payments over this time.

Dental insurance

Although more and more dental insurance plans now cover portions of orthodontic treatment, they often impose age limits. (Most plans cover orthodontic treatment only until the patient is sixteen years of age.) Get your dentist or orthodontist to submit an estimate to your insurance company before you begin treatment. That way you will have no unpleasant surprises.

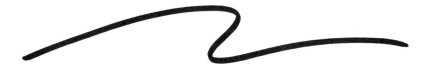

Treating gum disease (periodontics)

Periodontics is the branch of dentistry that is concerned with gums and their underlying tissues. Gums are the support system or foundation of the teeth. A house is only as good as its foundation — and teeth are only as healthy as their gums and supporting structures. Gum (periodontal) disease is the number one cause of tooth loss in adults. Nine out of ten people suffer from some form of gum disease at some point in their lives — and there's no need for it. Gum disease is *not* a sophisticated problem with mysterious causes. It's caused by plaque, plain and simple, and it can be prevented through regular, daily oral hygiene.

In the past, dentists paid little attention to the gums. Decay was so prevalent that filling teeth took up all of their time. When a tooth could no longer be filled it was extracted. But the advent of fluorides in drinking water has dramatically reduced the prevalence of decay. Better filling materials and restorative techniques mean that people keep their teeth longer. All of these improvements, plus concentrated research in periodontal disease, mean that more attention is being focussed on the health of gums.

A shocking sixty percent of the population suffers from some form of periodontal disease. It usually begins around the age of thirty-five. The most insidious thing about gum disease is that most people don't know they have it until it's almost too late. The reason? Periodontal disease is almost totally painless. So most people don't seek treatment until their teeth become loose and tender. Unfortunately most remedies only work in the early stages of the disease. Not much can be done at the loose tooth stage.

What is periodontal disease?

To understand periodontal disease, you need a brief lesson in dental anatomy.

The root of each of your teeth is embedded in bone. The tooth is connected to the bone by microscopic protein "strings." Millions of these strings anchor each tooth to the bone.

The bone around the teeth is covered by gum. Where gum meets each tooth it forms a little cuff around the

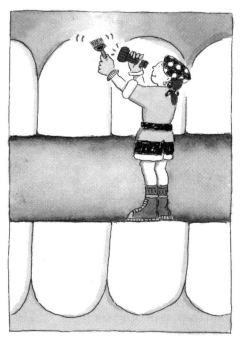

tooth. A tiny groove or crevice of gum exists around each tooth because of this cuff. It is at the bottom of this crevice that the gum is actually attached to the tooth. Normal, healthy gum has a crevice or groove less than three millimetres (one eighth of an inch) deep. This means that your toothbrush and floss can clean all plaque and bacteria from this crevice and everything is fine.

But if you *don't* brush and clean properly, you allow plaque to accumulate in this crevice. Plaque is a whitish, mushy, film-like substance that collects on teeth if they are not brushed regularly. It is a mixture of saliva, leftover food particles, and bacteria.

The longer plaque is left uncleaned in the gum crevice, the more it becomes a breeding ground for bacteria. In time this unremoved plaque hardens into calculus (tartar). Calculus is just calcified, hardened plaque.

Once calculus forms, it is not easily removed by brushing or flossing. Your dentist or hygienist must scale (scrape) it off your teeth. The trouble with calculus is that it provides microscopic nooks and crannies where more plaque and more bacteria can hide.

Certain types of bacteria in plaque and calculus produce waste products that irritate the surrounding gums. At first the gums become inflamed, reddish, and puffy; and they bleed easily. This stage of periodontal disease is called **gingivitis**. You can reverse the disease at this stage by removing plaque and calculus and their bacteria, thereby removing the bacterial waste products that irritate the gums.

If this is not done, periodontal disease progresses to the next stage. As more bacteria harbor in the calculus, which is becoming more plentiful, they produce more irritants and gums start to break down. Your body's immune system considers this bacterial attack an infection and sends out troops of special white blood cells to the area in an attempt to destroy the invading bacteria. The trouble is that in the process of destroying the bacteria, those blood cells also destroy some gum tissue. The crevice around the tooth gets deeper as gum is destroyed. As it gets deeper, it becomes virtually impossible to clean. This means that more plaque and bacteria are allowed to form unchecked in the deeper crevice. A vicious cycle is thus set up which sees more bacteria causing more immune response causing more destruction of gum, causing a still-deeper crevice. This deepened crevice is now called a pocket.

The pocket eventually becomes deep enough to be near the supporting bone and the millions of protein strings anchoring the tooth. Now the bacterial products and the immune system's response destroy not only gum tissues, they also destroy bone and protein strings. There is very little to hold the tooth in place once sufficient amounts of the bone and protein are destroyed. The tooth becomes loose, and is eventually lost as a result of periodontal disease.

Would I know if I had periodontal disease?

Unfortunately, periodontal disease is not painful. I say unfortunately because you would seek help early on if it was painful. Instead, most people notice some bleeding while brushing or flossing, and that's where it ends. Most people think that this is normal, or that they should stop flossing to help the situation. Stopping, of course, only leads to the formation of more plaque and bacteria in the gum crevice.

The bleeding seems to stop as this crevice gets deeper and becomes a pocket. This is because the infection is now deep in the pocket. Any bleeding may not be profuse enough to rise to the top of the pocket and be visible. In time, some of the gum no longer supported by bone will recede. But even at this stage most people assume that this recession is normal.

So you, the patient, have few if any signs of periodontal disease. However, be alert. Any bleeding during brushing should be reported to your dentist. As well, persistent bad breath or receding gums should be reported. These may be the only signs you notice. Any one, or combination, of the three is cause for concern.

How can my dentist tell if I have periodontal disease?

Even dentists often cannot tell if active periodontal disease is present. Periodontal disease is sporadic. This means that only a few teeth may be involved at any time. It also goes through active and passive stages. A lot of destruction of gum tissues may be going on, and then it may cease for months.

Dentists measure the depth of the crevice around each tooth on a regular basis and watch for areas that bleed easily during these measurements. The latter may indicate areas of active disease. Dentists also observe the color, shape, and tone of gums around all teeth. Taking periodic X-rays will also clearly show progressive bone destruction. These steps, taken together, should provide a good indication of whether periodontal disease is present.

Some dentists take microscopic samples of plaque from the gum pocket. The presence of certain types of bacteria in these samples indicates the presence of periodontal disease.

The newest technique for discovering periodontal disease is a DNA probe. Samples are taken from different suspicious areas and sent to a laboratory. Very sophisticated equipment is used to find specific DNA signatures of bacteria known to cause periodontal disease. If these are present, they confirm a diagnosis of periodontal disease.

How is periodontal disease controlled?

Prevention is a must.

Ninety percent of the control of periodontal disease rests with you. I will go over some treatments that your dentist or periodontist may perform to help you, but I stress that your own behavior is the key.

This sounds like a pretty dramatic statement, but research and experience prove over and over that proper oral hygiene at home is an absolute must for the control of periodontal disease.

Proper home care will reduce the amount of plaque present, the amount of tartar forming, and the number of bacteria collecting around your teeth. Removing the causes of infection removes the need for response by your immune system. No response means no destruction of your gums and supporting tissues.

Proper home care

What should you do to prevent gum disease? Back to the basics: You must brush your teeth thoroughly and meticulously, morning and night. And floss daily in-between all teeth. It never fails to amaze me how many people brush three to four times daily, but floss only once or twice a week at best. Obviously, these are motivated people who understand the reasons for proper care, but who think of flossing as something extra that isn't as necessary.

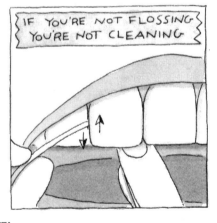

The best way I know to change this erroneous perception about flossing is to describe it like this: Brushing only cleans the cheek, tongue, and top surfaces of each tooth. The two surfaces of each tooth where teeth meet are not cleaned by brushing. The *only* way to clean these surfaces is by flossing. You clean forty percent of your tooth's surface only occasionally if you floss only occasionally. Thus a little more than half of the tooth surface in your mouth gets cleaned daily, and the rest gets cleaned once or twice a week — or less. What's even worse is that the sides that you do clean with brushing are kept fairly clean by your tongue and cheeks anyway. It is the areas in-between your teeth that are not being cleaned by anything, unless you floss. So the moral is this: If you don't floss, you're not really cleaning your teeth. You're just kidding yourself.

This sermon usually gets my patients motivated.

Regular checkups and cleanings

I said above that ninety percent of the fight against gum disease depends on you. The other ten percent is up to your dentist. Regular professional cleaning and scaling of your teeth is a must. For most people, regular means every six months. During this visit, your dentist will remove the calculus (tartar) that has formed on your teeth, and assess your gums for areas that bleed easily or are reddish, puffy, or otherwise inflamed. All of these are early signs of trouble that you may not be able to see yourself.

Once the problem areas are recognized, they will need a return visit to the dentist's office for a meticulous cleaning. You may require cleaning and monitoring visits every two to three months once the problems are brought under control. Twice yearly cleanings may not be sufficient for you at this stage. But again, at the risk of sounding repetitive, let me stress that your home care is still the key. Even if you are seeing a hygienist every two months, you still have to brush and floss meticulously at home every day.

Anti-microbial therapy

In some cases, frequent cleanings are not enough to reduce the bacterial populations in the pockets around your teeth. Medications may then be necessary to kill off some of the offending bacteria. These medications can be taken in tablet form, and are usually antibiotics, such as tetracycline.

Your dentist or periodontist may prescribe some rinses for you to use at home, too. The trouble with rinses is that they do not get far enough into the pockets to reach the offending bacteria. Your hygienist may use a special irrigating machine to flush out these pockets with an anti-microbial solution. You may also be given instructions on how to use special attachments for your water irrigator to flush out some of these pockets yourself.

The gums get a chance to heal once the levels of bacteria are down. Your continued home care will keep the bacteria controlled at low levels.

Gum surgery

Sometimes all of the above methods are not enough to keep periodontal disease under control. The reason for this is that the pockets have become too deep for you to keep clean. They may be so deep that the hygienist is unable to access the roots to remove the calculus. As you know by now, periodontal disease will continue if bacteria are allowed to collect around the roots. The solution is to surgically reduce the depth of these pockets. There are two ways of doing this.

In some cases, it is possible to expose the pockets, clean them and then fill them with certain natural or synthetic bonelike substances. The new substance fills up the pockets when they heal, and reduces their depth.

In other cases, it is not possible to do this. In these cases the dentist must expose the pockets, clean them again, and then remove some gum tissue from the top of the pockets. This, of course, makes the pockets shallower, but it also exposes the roots of the teeth. Exposed roots are only a small problem, and mostly a cosmetic one at that. However, if they are exposed at the front of the mouth, they may detract from your smile. Periodontists have an old saying for situations like this: "Better to have your teeth look longer than to have your teeth no longer."

If you want the cosmetic problem fixed, you can have the necessary teeth crowned (capped) in such a way that the crowns cover the exposed roots. Needless to say, this is a last resort. We try everything possible to prevent this from happening in the first place.

Again, as with all other treatment, home care after the surgery must be continued permanently. If you don't follow up at home, you may find that your newly-reduced pockets get deeper again — and you will be right back where you started. Pocket-reduction surgery gives you a second chance you can't afford to blow.

How long does periodontal treatment last?

The length of active periodontal treatment varies. Some people respond well after a couple of scaling appointments. They are also motivated enough to follow up with meticulous home care. For these cases, treatment can be quite short. Others may go the full distance, including periodontal surgery. They may be in treatment six to eighteen months. Home care is very critical — the final length of treatment depends on how motivated you are about keeping your teeth meticulously clean.

However, regular checkups and cleanings are a must even after the disease has been brought under control. These may have to be more frequent than the usual six months. As well, you cannot let up on your home care at any time.

To sum up: The bad news is that periodontal disease may return again. The good news is that through proper home care and proper maintenance *you* can control it.

Fees

Fees depend on the length and type of treatment required. Scaling appointments range from $120 to $160 per hour. Checkup visits are thirty-five to seventy dollars per visit. Surgery ranges from $200 to $3000 depending on how many teeth or areas are involved.

Most insurance plans cover you for these treatments although some have annual limits on scaling appointments. Your dentist or periodontist can submit an estimate to your insurance company to find out the extent of your coverage.

My regular dentist or a periodontist?

As with most branches of dentistry, this is a tricky question. Many dentists are very conscious of periodontal disease. They have acquired extended knowledge through courses and seminars. They may have specialized equipment such as microscopes to help them monitor a patient's progress. These dentists are quite capable of treating your gums right through the surgery phase. Most dentists, however, refer pockets over five to six millimetres to a periodontist. They will also refer any advanced cases that are not responding to their own treatment.

Once the patients are finished with active treatment, they usually return to their family dentist for regular maintenance. Some periodontists, however, insist on seeing their former patients for checkups and cleanings. Others alternate — that is, every other appointment is with the specialist, and the rest are with the family dentist.

You should see your family dentist at least every six months for a cavity check no matter what your periodontal maintenance regimen is. There's no use having great gums and decaying teeth, would't you agree?

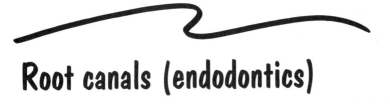

Root canals (endodontics)

The words **root canal** may be the most chilling in a dentist's vocabulary. When I tell new patients that they need a root canal, they seem to feel as if life as they know it has just ended. I can see it in their eyes. The way they sink down in their chair. "No! Please say it isn't so!" their body language says. Yet on the visit following root-canal treatment, ninety percent of my patients say there was nothing to it. Every time I do a root canal, I give the patient a prescription for some painkillers and instructions to get it filled only if necessary. Nine times out of ten, the patient never bothers to fill it.

So what is it about the words root canal that scare the dickens out of everyone? I think it's just ignorance. People have visions of the nerve of the tooth being tampered with. They think gums need to be cut, major surgery performed, the whole nine yards. *None* of this happens, as you will learn in this section. You will learn that root canals are a practical, viable means to keeping a damaged tooth and to using it as naturally as you would any other healthy tooth.

What is a root canal?

A root canal involves the removal of the infected or diseased tissues (parts) from the centre of the tooth. To better understand this, you will require a brief lesson in dental anatomy.

A tooth consists of two main parts. The hard, bony outer shell makes up the visible crown and the root of the tooth. Inside this shell is a hollow space. It is in this space that the nerves and blood vessels of the tooth reside. Together these are called soft tissues, and they make up the second major part of the tooth. The hollow space where the soft tissues reside is shaped like a chamber in the crown part of the tooth, and continues as a canal down each root of the tooth. At the tip of each root there is a small opening. The nerves and blood vessels exit and enter the tooth through this small opening, and connect with the nerves and the blood vessels of the jaw.

When the soft tissues inside the tooth become infected or diseased, they must be removed. This can be done in two ways. One is to extract the whole tooth. That way you get rid

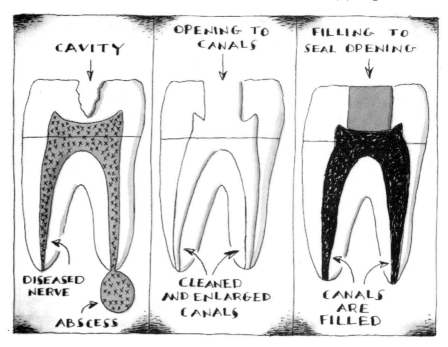

CAVITY

DISEASED NERVE

ABSCESS

OPENING TO CANALS

CLEANED AND ENLARGED CANALS

FILLING TO SEAL OPENING

CANALS ARE FILLED

of the diseased soft tissues inside the tooth. Unfortunately, you also get rid of the rest of the tooth. The better way is to remove the diseased soft tissues only, but to leave the hard shell of the tooth in place. This way, you keep your tooth and can continue to use it as you always did.

Who performs a root canal?

Root canal treatments have been part of the general dentistry curriculum at dental schools for about thirty–five years. As is the case with most specialties in dentistry, some dentists enjoy root canal work and others find it difficult and time-consuming. And even dentists who are skilled in this specialty may come up against a particularly difficult tooth that they do not wish to tackle. Enter the endodontist. He or she is the root canal specialist who will take on those difficult problems.

For some reason, patients are often reluctant to go to a specialist for a root canal treatment. They are used to their own dentists and they trust them. When I try to refer a patient to an endodontist they often say something along the lines of, "Doctor, you did my wife's root canal and she was okay. Why don't you go ahead and do mine too?" Don't put your dentist under pressure like that. If your dentist feels that a specialist is required, he or she usually has a pretty good reason. Ask what it is and then follow the advice.

How is the root canal performed?

The offending tooth is frozen. A small opening is made on the top, chewing part of the tooth. If we are dealing with a front tooth, we make the opening on the tongue side of the tooth where it won't be seen. The opening is extended to the hollow centre of the tooth, where the diseased soft tissues are. Each canal in every root is cleaned out right to the tip. Then the hollow space in the centre of the tooth and all the canals leading to it are filled with a rubber-like material. The initial opening is closed with a filling and the root canal treatment is over and done with.

Is there any discomfort after the root canal is finished?

In some cases, you may experience some discomfort for a day or two following the root canal treatment. Many patients find this puzzling. "But doctor, didn't you take all the nerves out?" is the usual question. The answer is, of course, yes. But the discomfort you feel is not from the tooth itself. It's from the bone surrounding the tooth. The simple action of cleaning and instrumenting the tooth may set up a mild, temporary inflammation in the bone surrounding the tooth. This will clear in a couple of days. Anti-inflammatory medications such as aspirin or Motrin are best for this mild discomfort.

My friend had a root canal and needed a number of appointments. Why?

A root canal treatment should ideally be performed when the abscess is small, before a full-blown infection has set into the tooth. It may not be possible to complete the root canal in one appointment once the infection is extensive and there is a lot of swelling in the area. Several appointments may be necessary to drain all of the infection from the tooth.

This is why you should have the problem tooth treated as soon as your dentist tells you to do so. Putting it off will only lead to a worse infection in the tooth and to more problems during treatment.

If the tooth is infected, why can't it be healed with an antibiotic?

Good question. For an infection in any other part of the body, simple antibiotics would suffice. But a root canal is necessary if there is infection in a tooth. Why?

Because teeth are different. Here's why: If, for example, your finger becomes infected, it becomes reddish and swollen. This is because your immune system sends extra blood into the infected area. This extra blood carries special white blood cells that fight the infection. Your finger

can accommodate the swelling, because the skin covering it
is elastic.

Your immune system tries to do the same thing if a tooth
becomes infected. It tries to rush extra blood and bacteria-
fighting white cells into the tooth. However, unlike the skin
on your finger, the hard shell of the tooth can't expand or
swell to accommodate this extra blood. The sudden increase in blood flow squeezes all the blood vessels inside the
tooth and chokes off all blood circulation — the opposite of
what should happen. This lack of circulation causes the soft
tissues inside the tooth, including blood vessels and nerves,
to die. Once dead, these decomposing tissues are a perfect
breeding ground for bacteria, which turn this mess into
pus. More and more pus forms and cannot be contained in
the tooth. Some of it is pushed out the openings at the end
of the root tips, forming little sacks of pus in the jaw bone at
the end of the root. This is what is called an **abscess**. The
build-up of pressure on this abscess causes the pain of an
abscessed tooth. At this point, antibiotics may control the
abscess in the bone to a certain extent. However, since
blood is not circulating in the tooth, it cannot carry the
antibiotic into the tooth to kill the bacteria. So more pus
forms in the tooth and goes back out into the abscess in the
bone. The only way to stop this process is to physically clean
out the canals in the tooth. This is what a root canal
procedure does.

Is the tooth as good as new after the root canal?

The root canal treatment gets rid of the infection in the
tooth. It does not bring circulation — and, thus, life — back
to the tooth. The tooth tends to become dry and more
brittle than a normal tooth due to lack of circulation. This
is why a root canal-treated tooth must be restored with a
crown (cap), or at least an onlay type of restoration, to hold
the sides of the tooth together and prevent breaking or
cracking.

Patients who need root canal treatment sometimes tell
me stories about a friend or relative who had one and how
the tooth subsequently fell apart and was lost. This only

means that a proper restoration such as a crown or onlay was not placed on the tooth after the root canal treatment. When a proper restoration is put in place, it makes the tooth as strong and durable as any untreated tooth.

Costs

The fee for a root canal varies, depending on how many roots and, therefore, how many canals, a tooth has. A front tooth with only one canal will cost $250 to $350 to treat. A back molar tooth with three or four canals will cost $450 to $550. These fees are for the root canal treatment only and do not include the final crown restoration.

Most insurance plans consider root canal treatment a basic type of service. You will usually be reimbursed at the same rate as you would be for regular fillings and cleanings.

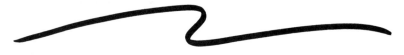

Oral surgery

Oral surgery deals with the extraction (removal) of teeth, including wisdom teeth. It also covers surgical jaw repairs and reconstructions of jaws damaged in accidents (frequently automobile accidents). Oral surgeons also repair birth defects and perform cosmetic and orthodontic surgery involving jawbones.

Extractions

In the old days of dentistry, teeth were either filled or pulled. Those were the only choices available. As a result, it was common for people over the age of forty to be left with unsightly gaps where their teeth used to be.

Nowadays many more choices are available. Root canals, gum treatments, and advanced restorative procedures, such as crowns and bonding, allow us to keep teeth which were previously considered hopeless.

In today's dentistry, few teeth are extracted. Teeth are taken out only if they are hopelessly destroyed, if they endanger the health of remaining teeth, or if they cannot be treated because of poor health or financial difficulties.

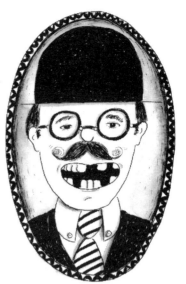

What to do after an extraction

If you have a tooth extracted, make sure you follow your dentist's instructions for home care.

In general, you should bite on a bundle of gauze for ten to fifteen minutes after a tooth is extracted. The pressure will help stop the initial bleeding and will allow a blood clot to form. You should not leave the dental office until all bleeding has stopped. The dentist or oral surgeon will give you some gauze to take home. If any bleeding occurs later at home, it can be stopped if you again bite on some gauze for ten to fifteen minutes. Don't be alarmed by seeing a lot of blood in your mouth. A few drops of blood mixed with your saliva looks like a flood, but in fact it's nearly all saliva. Don't panic.

If painkillers have been prescribed, they should be taken before all of the freezing wears off. That way, they will already be working when the freezing is gone and your discomfort will be greatly reduced.

During the first twenty-four hours after an extraction, try to take it easy. Strain and exercise may lead to renewed bleeding from the extraction site.

Eat soft foods and don't chew above the extraction socket. Avoid smoking. Nicotine interferes with blood-clot formation. Avoid alcohol, too, because it will react with the painkillers and cause potentially serious overdose reactions. **Do** drink lots of fluids such as juices and water.

If any swelling develops, it will be within seventy-two hours of the extraction. As you feel the swelling coming on, apply an ice pack for twenty minutes at a time, every half hour to an hour. Once you see that the swelling has stopped increasing, apply a heating pad to reduce it. Again, no more than twenty minutes at a time, every half hour to an hour. This will help resolve the swelling faster.

After the first twenty-four hours, rinse your mouth with salt and water. A solution of one teaspoon of salt in two-thirds of a glass of warm water is ideal. Rinse three to five times a day. Try to keep your mouth as clean as possible. Keep brushing the remaining teeth as best you can, but don't try to brush around the extraction site until all soreness is gone.

After an extraction, the socket where the tooth used to be heals from the bottom up. This means that it may be several months before the site feels completely even.

Wisdom Teeth

As humans continue to evolve, their jaws seem to be getting smaller. **Wisdom teeth** are the last teeth to erupt into the mouth. They are also called third molars, because they are the third molar tooth in the mouth. Normally there are four of them, one in each corner of the mouth. There is nothing unusual or mystical about them, aside from the fact that they erupt between the ages of sixteen and twenty years.

Because wisdom teeth are the last to come in, they may not have enough room to erupt into proper position. Because of this, one of the following may happen.

● **They may become fully impacted.**
In this position, one or all of the wisdom teeth are physically prevented from erupting into the mouth. They are usually forced to grow at an angle where they hit the roots of the teeth in front of them. Alternatively, they may be pointing down, forward, or even backward instead of straight up. Fully-impacted teeth will never erupt on their own. Your dentist or oral surgeon must decide if your fully-impacted teeth are causing any damage. Some may be left alone, and X-rayed every three to five years to ensure that there are no cysts or other growths forming around them. Others may be pushing or damaging the roots of the teeth in front of them. In this situation, they should be extracted.

● **They may be partly impacted.**
In this situation, the wisdom tooth is partly erupted into the mouth. However, it is lodged behind the tooth in front of it or behind some bone in a way that prevents further eruption. This tooth should be extracted. The reason for this is that gum does not attach properly to a partly erupted tooth. The result is a pouch of loose gum around the wisdom tooth where plaque and food accumulate and cause infection.

● **They may be fully erupted but dislocated.**
In this scenario, the wisdom tooth is fully erupted into the mouth. However, because of a lack of room in the jaw, the tooth is pushed to the side of the jaw, usually toward the cheek. Teeth in this position serve no function, because they don't bite against anything. They are difficult to keep clean. As a result they frequently develop cavities and localized gum infections. They should be extracted so that the teeth and gums in front of them can be kept clean and healthy.

Should I have all four wisdom teeth extracted?

Sometimes only one or two wisdom teeth will fall into one of the above categories. Usually it is the bottom wisdom teeth that run out of room. To decide if the other wisdom tooth should be retained, your dentist will examine your bite. If a wisdom tooth is in a good, cleanable position, and is biting against another tooth, it can be left in place. Both teeth should be extracted if extracting a poorly positioned tooth will leave the opposing tooth without anything to bite against.

Who should extract my wisdom teeth?

If the teeth are fully or mostly erupted, they can be extracted by your family dentist. Fully impacted wisdom teeth are best left to an oral surgeon. Oral surgeons are dentists who have spent an additional four to five years of training in oral surgery. As they spend much of their time extracting impacted wisdom teeth, they are your best bet for this procedure.

Oral surgeons are able to administer general anesthesia, as well. So your extractions can be done while you are asleep.

Can there be complications from wisdom teeth extractions?

Most complications are just magnified consequences of any extraction. There may be a lot of swelling, bruising, and discomfort following the surgery if a lot of work has been necessary to reach the impacted tooth.

Dry sockets, which can occur in any extraction, occur more commonly with wisdom teeth. A dry socket condition means that the initial blood clot got dislodged or never formed properly. This could happen through chewing, spitting, brushing, or smoking. Without the blood clot, the body has no scaffolding on which to heal the area.

If you are experiencing severe pain several days after the extraction, have your dentist or oral surgeon check for dry sockets. If you have one, you will have a self-dissolving sponge placed in the socket to provide the scaffolding needed for proper healing.

Replacing teeth (prosthodontics)

Prosthodontics is a specialty of dentistry that deals with the replacement of missing or lost teeth. There are two ways to replace missing teeth. The first method involves a **fixed prosthesis**, which replaces teeth permanently and cannot be removed. The second involves a **removable prosthesis**, such as a set of dentures, which the patient can easily take out.

When do teeth need to be replaced?

Drifting teeth

The teeth in your jaw are like stones in an old-fashioned archway: they all support each other. Taking one out may not cause an immediate collapse of the arch, but it will put more stress on the remaining stones, which will eventually loosen and fall out, too. It's the same with teeth. They tend to drift or move, when one tooth is removed, until they touch another tooth. Usually front teeth move toward the back, and back teeth move toward the front.

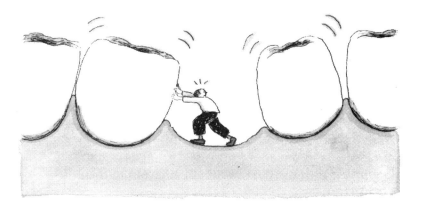

If a tooth is lost, it leaves a space, and the two teeth on either side of it move slowly and inexorably into that space. The entire tooth moves, roots and all. As a result, spaces are opened up between these teeth and their neighbors. In time the next set of neighboring teeth move also, opening more spaces further down the line. Food gets packed into these spaces, and pushes the gums down along the roots of the teeth.

Eventually an inflammation sets in, which in time leads to periodontal disease. Angular spaces form around the tilted teeth and plaque accumulates in these spaces, because they are hard to reach with a brush. Eventually the gums become inflamed and recede, which weakens the underlying support of these teeth.

As teeth shift and drift, they begin to lean. The force of your bite is no longer directed straight up and down the long axis of your teeth. This means that from now on, every time you bite you are pushing your teeth at more and more of an angle, which will eventually loosen them.

All this movement, gum recession, and so on, soon starts to affect your bite. The far side of the leaning tooth is now higher than the surrounding teeth. This means that as you chew, you hit this tooth first, and hardest, with every bite. This further weakens the support of the tooth. The constant pounding may cause so much stress that the nerves and vessels inside the tooth are damaged and the tooth becomes abscessed.

The continual striking of this raised corner of the tooth causes a great deal of pain. Your brain, reacting to avoid the pain, tries to intervene and tell your jaw to change its pattern of closing. This in turn may lead to problems in the jaw joints (see TMJ Syndrome, pages 174 –178).

Studies conducted over an extended period of time show that the two teeth surrounding the space where a tooth has been lost are the most likely to be lost next. Now *three* teeth are lost — and the above process continues relentlessly, beginning with the next two teeth adjacent to the now enlarged space.

Overgrowing teeth

Since teeth erupt (grow) out of the jawbone until they hit something, they will continue to grow if there are no opposing teeth. Eventually the root portion of a tooth that erupts like this becomes exposed. Naturally, this may make that tooth very sensitive, particularly to cold. If it is a multi-rooted tooth, it may eventually overgrow to such a degree that the dividing point of the roots is above the gum instead of below the gum as it should be. This creates an area that is very difficult to keep clean. Plaque and bacteria congregate and cause severe destruction of the supporting gum and bone. The tooth loosens and is eventually lost.

There is more: The overgrown tooth now sticks out above the line of all the other teeth. Your jaw moves from side to side when you chew, and the opposing teeth around the missing tooth hit the overgrown tooth. This further adds to the loosening of the overgrown tooth, and puts stress on the opposing teeth that hit it. Again, your jaw attempts to avoid this interference. This avoidance puts stress on the jaw joints and on the muscles controlling the bite. Eventually this may lead to TMJ problems.

In time, the overgrown tooth falls out due to weakened support, and the vicious cycle starts again, beginning with the two teeth on either side of the lost tooth.

Now you can see how a single missing tooth can lead to the loss of many other teeth. How can you avoid this? You can avoid it by replacing a lost tooth as soon as possible.

Fixed prostheses

Bridges

The best way to replace missing teeth is to use **fixed bridges**. A bridge, just as its name implies, bridges the gap between teeth. It is permanently attached to existing teeth on either side of the gap where teeth are missing. There are several types of bridges.

● **Conventional bridges**
Conventional bridges are head and shoulders ahead of other types of bridges. They are by far the most widely used and most reliable kind of bridge. The tooth or teeth on either side of the gap are prepared just as they would be for a crown (cap). About one to one-and-a-half millimetres of tooth is removed all around. An impression (mold) is taken of the prepared teeth. The laboratory makes a metal bridge based on the model made from this impression. The bridge consists of crowns (caps) for the prepared teeth. Attached between these crowns are the artificial teeth that will fill the existing gap. All these metal teeth (crowns and the false teeth in-between them) are covered with a porcelain finish that matches the color of the patient's remaining teeth. When the bridge returns from the laboratory, it is cemented (glued) over the existing, prepared teeth. Once cemented, the bridge cannot be removed. It is just like the patient's own teeth. It doesn't rock or wiggle, and it is used and cared for just as if it were a set of natural teeth.

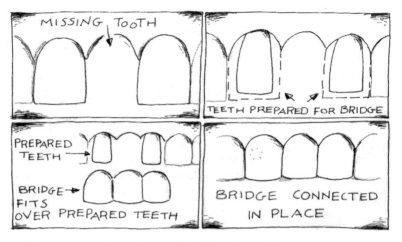

This conventional type of bridge has a life expectancy of fifteen to twenty years. Many last much longer with proper home care.

Because the teeth on either side of the gap are crowned (capped), they are strengthened as well.

The cost of a bridge like this depends on the number of teeth being crowned and the number of teeth being replaced. Each crowned tooth costs $600-$700, and each replacement tooth is $400 to $500. The smallest possible bridge replacing one missing tooth and crowning two teeth (one on either side of the gap) will cost $1600 to $1900.

● **Bonded bridges**

Sometimes the teeth on either side of the gap created by the missing tooth are healthy teeth with no large restorations (fillings). Some people don't like the idea of putting crowns on teeth like these since those teeth don't need to be strengthened. These teeth may be good candidates for **bonding**. To create a **bonded bridge**, the laboratory makes a false tooth with wing-like attachments on either side. These attachments are then bonded onto the adjacent teeth to hold the false tooth in place. The wings can be made of metal or porcelain. If they're made of porcelain, they can be veneered (see pages 97–100) to blend with the adjacent teeth.

Bonding works well when there is not much stress on the bridge. But there is always a chance that the bridge will come loose. It can be rebonded, but it will never be as secure as a conventional bridge.

The current fee for a bonded bridge in which a single tooth is replaced is $800 to $1400.

Implants

A **dental implant** is a device that can be anchored to the jawbone where no natural teeth exist and to which prosthetic (false) teeth, can be attached.

The use of implants is one of the fastest growing areas of dentistry. Implants have flexible and diverse uses and can be used in an amazing variety of situations — everything from restoring single missing teeth to reconstructing mouths where no natural teeth are present. Right now only ten to fifteen percent of dentists do implants. Over the next ten years, the percentage is sure to rise rapidly.

Just about anyone who is missing one or more teeth is a candidate for implants. When dentists first started placing implants, they were doing them only for desperate, full-denture wearers who couldn't stand wearing their dentures. The prevailing attitude was that this was the treatment of last resort — what could be lost by trying? Now, all that has changed, and implants have become an option in every tooth replacement situation. Patients with no natural teeth left in their mouth love implants because they make wearing dentures much easier and more enjoyable. People with missing back teeth like them because they obviate the need for removable partial dentures. Young people who have lost a single tooth due to an accident like them because no filing of adjacent, virgin teeth is necessary. All in all, implants have a varied and growing clientele.

History of implants
Implants aren't new. Dentists were using them as early as the 1920s. These early implants were usually large metal objects, shaped like flat blades, with all kinds of intricate patterns cut into them. They were either inserted into slots cut in the jawbone, or placed just under the gum on top of the jawbone.

The trouble with these early implants was that if they failed — which they did, frequently — they often destroyed a lot of bone in the process. If a person had a hard time wearing dentures before the implant was placed, that person could find denture-wearing impossible after a failed implant. Because of these risks, implants were considered a last-resort treatment for people without any natural teeth who were unable to wear dentures anyway.

In the 1960s, a Swedish researcher named P.I. Branemark began studying implant methods. The implants we use today are the result of Branemark's studies. Branemark found that the best implants were made of a Titanium alloy. They were small cylinders measuring three to five millimetres across and seven to seventeen millimetres long, containing many holes, nooks, and crannies for bone to grow into.

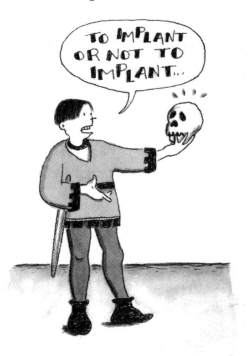

How are implants placed?
There are 3 stages to implant treatment.

● **Making the decision**
Implants work well in many different situations, but they are not a panacea for every problem. It is imperative that your dentist sit down with you and explain any possible drawbacks or limitations of implants for your particular situation.

You must also understand that placing an implant is a six to twelve month procedure involving many appointments and several surgical treatments. Are you fully prepared for this commitment of time and energy?

And last, but crucially important as always, implants demand meticulous oral hygiene once they are placed. Are you prepared to invest the extra time and effort?

Most implant patients do claim that it's all worth it in the end. But you should know what you are getting into ahead of time.

● **Planning an implant**

Once both you and your dentist are sure that implants are for you, the two of you must study X-rays and models to decide how many and what kind of implants you need, and where they will be placed. You also must choose what type of false tooth (prosthesis) will go over the implant.

● **Surgical placement of an implant**

The surgical placement of an implant or implants in your jawbone may be done by your dentist, an oral surgeon, or a periodontist. Any one of these professionals may be qualified through special courses to perform this operation.

Here's how an implant is placed. First, the jaw is anesthetized. If you wish, you may be put completely to sleep for this. The surgeon then makes an opening in the bone, places the implant, and sutures (stitches) the site.

Next comes the healing process, which takes three to nine months. During this time, bone grows tightly all around the implant and the entire implant is literally buried in your jawbone. None of the implant is visible in your mouth by the time healing is complete. The implant is not used for anything during this time.

The dentist who placed the implant then removes the gum that has grown over the implant, thus exposing the tip of the implant. Then he or she screws into the implant a healing collar made of plastic or metal. This healing collar sticks out one to two millimeters over your gums. This is the first time you see any part of your implant in your mouth.

You wear the healing collar for three to four weeks until the gum around it is healed and healthy. Then it's time to see the dentist who will place the false tooth. This may or may not be your own dentist, depending on whether or not he or she does implants.

This is the last phase of treatment. The dentist unscrews the healing collars and the final posts or attachments are screwed into the implants. Impressions (molds) are taken, and the laboratory makes the final "prosthesis," which may be a single crown (cap), a bridge, or a denture.

Are there any reasons not to have implants?
Yes. If you suffer from any bone disease — osteoporosis, for example — you are not a good implant candidate. Specific mouth conditions may also rule out implants. For example, much of the bony ridge in your jaw has probably been resorbed if your teeth have been missing for a long time and there may not be enough bone left for implants. Or, the area of bone where you require an implant may contain major blood vessels or nerves, which may make implant placement risky. This is often the case when replacing back teeth on the lower jaw. On the back of the upper jaw, your sinuses may be very close to the ridge of the jawbone, making implants inadvisable. The width and height of the bone present is also a consideration.

You must be psychologically prepared for the surgery, too. This is no small matter. Treatment will probably take six to twelve months or even longer. Are you a patient enough patient for this?

What kinds of restorations are possible with implants?
Implants cover the whole range from simple tooth replacement to complete mouth rehabilitation.

Replacing a single tooth with an implant
If only one tooth is missing you can replace it with a fixed bridge. But unless you settle for a bonded bridge (see pages 160 –161) — which is not as secure as a fixed bridge — you will have to have the adjacent teeth crowned (capped). However, you may be reluctant to have these teeth crowned if they are virgin (have no restorations at all). Getting a single implant allows you to replace a single tooth without touching the adjacent teeth.

Replacing several teeth with implants
If several teeth are missing, they can be replaced with two or more implants. These make a base for a fixed bridge which will replace the missing teeth. This bridge is permanent and does not have to be attached to any remaining natural teeth.

Rehabilitating an entire mouth with implants
When no natural teeth are present in the jaw, several
options are available.

● **Option 1:** Five or six implants are placed. A fixed bridge
replacing ten to twelve teeth — or pretty well all your teeth
in that jaw — is attached to these implants. A fixed bridge
such as this feels solid and acts just like your own teeth.

● **Option 2:** Five or six implants are placed. A special bar is
attached to these implants and a denture is made to fit over
this bar. This attachment is very secure and feels very snug.
It has the advantage of allowing you to remove the denture
for cleaning. As well, only the bar is attached to the implants, so it's easier to keep them clean as well.

● **Option 3:** If, for anatomic or financial reasons, placing so
many implants is not possible, the dentist will place only two
implants. Then a denture, with snap-like attachments on
the implants and the underside of the denture is made.
This kind of denture still rests on your gums but it is held
securely in place by the snap attachments.

Costs
The cost of implants is comparable to that of other prosthetic devices. For example: replacing a single tooth with an
implant costs $1500 to $1900. This is roughly equivalent to
the cost of a bridge replacing the same tooth.

Multi-tooth replacements proportionately cost more. The
cost usually runs at approximately $1000 per implant and
$400 to $700 per replacement tooth. So a full jaw reconstruction with five implants and ten fixed teeth would cost
around $10,000. A five-implant removable denture would
be $6000 to $7000. A two-implant setup with a denture
would cost aproximately $3000 to $3500.

Because implants are fairly new, they are not covered by
most insurance companies. This situation will probably
change as the treatment becomes more established.

Removable prostheses

Dentures

Dentists call dentures **"removable prosthodontics."** A **partial denture** replaces a few missing teeth. A **full denture** replaces all of the teeth in one or both jaws.

Partial dentures

Partial dentures, sometimes known as **partial bridges**, replace missing teeth, and are attached to existing teeth by clasps. Partial dentures are a reasonably economical alternative to permanent tooth replacements such as bridges or implants. They are especially useful when all the back teeth are missing. A bridge cannot be made in such a situation because there are no teeth to which a bridge can be anchored. One partial denture will fill all the spaces left when teeth are missing in several areas of the jaw. Several bridges would be required to fill the same spaces, and would cost a great deal more.

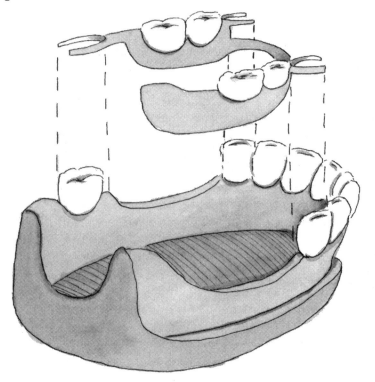

How are partial dentures made?

Partial dentures are custom-made to fit your mouth. First, your dentist takes an impression of your upper and lower teeth in order to study their position, alignment, and bite. Then the dentist designs the optimum type of denture. The X-rays of your teeth are used to decide how many clasps will be necessary, which teeth will support the denture, and which teeth it will be attached to. Factors such as aesthetics, ability to clean around the denture, and stress on existing teeth are all considered.

Your next appointment may involve some minor adjustments (filing) of your teeth. This is done to reduce interferences with your denture, as well as to allow for better attachment of the denture to your teeth. A new impression is taken of the prepared teeth. The laboratory then casts a metal framework for the denture. The false teeth are attached to this framework. After you've had a couple of "try-in" appointments, you're ready to use your new partial denture.

Metal or plastic?

I mentioned above that your partial denture is cast out of metal. Some partials are made solely from plastic. They cost a bit less but frankly, I don't think they're worth the savings. They take an inordinate toll on the health of your remaining teeth and gums. Cast metal partials, in contrast, have rests that prevent the denture from stripping gum from your tooth during chewing. They also have guides that support and stabilize your existing teeth. Plastic dentures have neither.

And because metal is stronger, it makes a denture that is lighter and less bulky than a plastic one. So unless you truly cannot afford them, I strongly recommend cast metal partials.

Should I wear my partials all the time?

No. You should remove your partials at night. Wearing them twenty-four hours a day is like wearing your shoes around the clock. Your feet need a chance to breathe. So do your gums. Constant pressure of the partial on the ridges between your teeth prevents proper circulation in the gums in these areas. As well, constant contact with plastic leads to reddish, irritated gums. Constant wearing of your dentures will produce gum soreness and a foul odour, and, over many years, may lead to growths and tumors. Three good reasons to remove them at night!

Removing your dentures at night gives your gums a rest. It may take a few minutes in the morning before your dentures settle in, but at least your gums will be healthier.

Can denture clasps cause cavities or wear out my teeth?

No. This is an old wives' tale. Some people are convinced that denture clasps around their natural teeth cause decay in these areas. Trust me on this: bacteria in plaque is the *only* thing that causes decay. If you are keeping your teeth and denture clean, you are removing plaque and reducing bacteria, thereby preventing decay.

One part of this old wives' tale is true, however: the additional hardware of dentures, clasps, and so on, creates more nooks and crannies where plaque can harbor. This means that you must be doubly vigilant about your oral hygiene.

How do I clean my teeth and my partials?

Because partial dentures are removable, they must be taken out each time you clean your teeth. Once you have taken out the partial, brush and floss your teeth as always. Then, using a regular toothbrush and soap, thoroughly clean your partial denture. Clean around the false teeth, under the denture, and around all clasps. Fill your sink with a couple of inches of water when you're cleaning your denture. That way, if it slips out of your hands it will hit water, not the sink. Always keep your denture in water or within a wet towel when it's not in your mouth. The plastic may warp if the denture dries out and this will alter the denture's fit.

If you are conscientious with your cleaning, you shouldn't have to use cleaning tablets and powders. If you do choose a cleanser, make sure you get one that is compatible with metal partials. Some of the older products could corrode the metal.

Do I have to wear my dentures regularly?

Teeth are always drifting and moving. Part of the reason for having a denture is to prevent teeth from drifting and tilting into the spaces left by missing teeth. If you only wear your dentures occasionally, you may eventually find that they no longer fit because substantial drifting has occurred in-between wearings. Occasional wear may also cause back and forth movements on your teeth that may lead to their loosening.

Full dentures

If you are missing all of your teeth in your upper or your lower jaw, you will have to wear full dentures.

What are full dentures?

A full denture is a removable prosthetic device used to replace all of the teeth in the upper or lower jaw. Full dentures are usually made of plastic, with false teeth set directly into the plastic base. Plastic bases, instead of metal, are used for full dentures because they are lighter and easier to add to during future relines. Unlike partial dentures, which are best made of metal, full dentures have no clasps to attach them to any existing teeth. Therefore, no metal is necessary.

In the upper jaw, the full denture covers the entire roof of the mouth. In the lower jaw, because of the tongue, the denture covers only the bony ridge of the jaw, and is shaped like a horseshoe.

What holds a full denture in place?

Full dentures are mostly held in place by a vacuum suction which forms under the denture and causes it to adhere to the gums of the jawbones. Additional suctional force is created by a film of moisture between the denture and gums. A well-designed denture also makes use of the tongue, the cheek muscles, and any bulges in the jawbone to hold the denture in place.

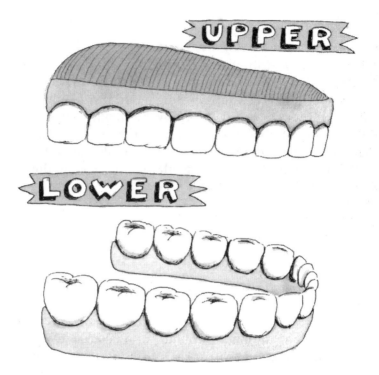

Are upper and lower dentures equally stable?
No. Upper dentures tend to be more stable than lower
dentures. Why? Because the upper denture has the entire
roof of the mouth against which to form suction. This
makes the upper denture fairly stable and secure. The lower
denture has very little surface to adhere to. Denture wearers, unless they have very large bony ridges along their
lower jaws, will find their full lower dentures very loose and
floppy.

So if you still have any lower teeth left at all and are
considering a full denture, you should, in my opinion, hang
onto whatever lower teeth you can. Over my years in dentistry, I have seen many patients with full lower dentures.
And I am not exaggerating when I say that ninety-five
percent of these full lower dentures are loose, floppy, and
agonizing to wear. The only relief for the wearers of these
dentures is implant treatment — assuming that their health
will allow it, and that they still have enough bone in their
lower jaw in which some implants can be placed.

How should I clean my dentures?

The best way to clean your dentures is with soap and water. If you do this consistently from the time your dentures are new, you should have no trouble keeping them clean for years. A specially designed, large denture brush is ideal for this. It looks just like a regular brush, but it is three times larger. The safest way to clean your dentures is to fill your basin with two to three inches of water and to clean your dentures over the basin. That way, should your dentures slip out of your hands, they won't be damaged or broken because the water will cushion the fall.

To keep your dentures looking like new, you should try to clean them after meals as often as possible. If, despite your best efforts, your dentures do build up some tartar, they can be placed by your dentist in an ultrasonic bath for a few minutes to remove the buildup.

Older, stained dentures will benefit from effervescent baths, which are available in any drugstore. Many people also like the fresh taste that these solutions leave on their dentures. Any of the commercial preparations available will do the job. However, *never* soak your dentures in regular bleach solution. The bleach will remove the coloring from the denture base as well as the sheen from the plastic teeth. The result is an unsightly denture that cannot be repaired and will have to be remade.

How often should I remove my dentures?

You should remove your dentures every night and keep them in water through the night. This allows your gums a chance to breathe. Wearing dentures around the clock is like wearing your shoes around the clock. Both your gums and your feet need some time to be free of the constraints and pressure of being enclosed in an artificial structure. Wearing dentures all the time leads to inflamed and some-times sore gums. Constant inflammation and irritation of this kind may lead to growth of tumors in the area.

Some people find that it is difficult to put dentures in in the morning after having taken them out at night. This period of adjustment rarely lasts more than fifteen to twenty minutes, and is due to a slight increase in volume, during the night, of your fresh and rejuvenated gums.

See your dentist for an adjustment if it takes longer than this to get readjusted to your dentures in the morning.

Do I need to see a dentist regularly if I have full dentures?

One of the most common misconceptions in dentistry is that once you have no natural teeth left, you never need to see a dentist again. This is simply not true. The bones and gums inside your mouth change constantly. A denture that fit very well when it was first made may not do so a few months or years later. Changes are gradual, however, so you may not realize that your dentures are not fitting as snugly as they did at first.

I insist that my denture patients visit me once a year. During these visits, I check for looseness and loss of stability in the denture; I check the way upper and lower teeth bite together; and I carefully examine the tongue, lips, cheeks, floor of the mouth, and all the soft tissues under the dentures.

What problems might I have if I don't see a dentist regularly?

The denture may rock from side to side or from front to back when bone support underneath it changes. This rocking dramatically speeds up further loss of bone under the denture. The edges of the denture dig deeper into the soft tissues of the cheeks when bone is lost. Because this digging happens so gradually, it may not cause much pain. But this low-level chronic irritation to the cheeks can cause the formation of growths and extra folds in these areas. Such growths have to be surgically removed because if they are left in place, they can turn cancerous.

You need a dentist, too, to determine whether you are removing your dentures often enough to prevent irritation to your gums. Gum irritations can turn cancerous, too, although this is rare.

For all these reasons, it is vital that you make your dentist your friend — even if you have lost all your natural teeth and you wear full dentures.

What are relines?

The underside of a full denture no longer fits very well as bones and gums change beneath it. This is because the denture was made to fit these areas before the changes occurred and, because the denture is made of plastic, it doesn't change as your mouth does.

This is where **relines** come in.

An impression (mold) is taken by filling the inside of your denture with soft impression material. Wherever the bones and gums have shrunk, there will be a thicker layer of the impression material left in the denture.

The laboratory then fills in these areas by substituting extra denture plastic for the impression material. The end result is that the underside of your denture once again exactly fits the bones and gums beneath it. You end up with a well-fitting, more retentive denture.

On average, you will need a reline every two to four years. Bottom dentures need to be relined more frequently than top dentures because bone disappears much faster in the bottom jaw than it does in the top one.

The average cost of a reline is $120 to $150. Relines are covered by dental insurance.

Denture adhesives

Many denture wearers resort to **denture adhesives** to help keep their dentures in place. Before you do this, have your dentist check your dentures first. Often the poor fit is a result of changes in your mouth and can be corrected by relining the denture.

In general, unless very little bone support is present, a well-fitting denture requires no adhesives to keep it in place.

TMJ Syndrome (Temporomandibular Joint Dysfunction Syndrome)

If you have pain or discomfort when you open or close your mouth, if you feel stiffness and soreness in your face or if you get frequent migraines, you may be a victim of TMJ Dysfunction Syndrome. TMJ Syndrome is a frustrating and debilitating condition. And it is one of the least understood areas in dentistry.

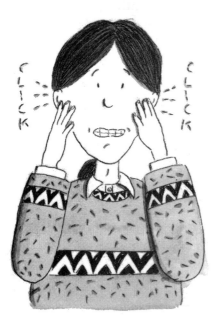

If you put your fingers on your face, just in front of your ears, and move your jaw up and down, you can feel the movement of your temporomandibular joints. They are like hinges connecting your lower jaw to your skull. These joints are unique among the joints in your body because of their sophisticated internal design, which enables them to slide forward and backward at the same time as they rotate to open your jaw.

They are further unique because, unlike any other joint, their final resting position is determined by hard contact between your upper and lower teeth. Think about it: All other joints — your knees or elbows, for example — come to rest when soft tissues, such as muscle tissues, meet. This creates flexibility and cushioning for the joint. Not so when the hard teeth of your upper and lower jaw meet.

Finally, your temporomandibular joints are unique because the left and right joints are solidly connected with each other through your lower jaw. You cannot move one without the other. So any stress caused by your bite on these joints will have to be accommodated by both the left and the right joint simultaneously. It is conceivable that *one* of the joints might manage to do so; but to expect both of them to do so together, in perfect harmony with each other, is asking a great deal. So it's not surprising that problems can develop.

It is because of all of these unique features that the TM joints are so difficult to understand and so difficult to treat when something goes wrong.

Signs and symptoms of TMJ Syndrome

Many dentists consider clicking or grinding noises from one or both of the TM joints to be signs of trouble brewing. I personally disagree with this. Many people go through life making the most bizarre noises with their joints and never miss a meal or a night's sleep. If you have noisy joints, by all means have your dentist check them. But don't rush into treatment unless you are experiencing pain or discomfort.

Warning signs of TMJ Syndrome:

● Pain or tenderness in the joints

● Inability to open the mouth fully

● Chronic stiffness or soreness in facial muscles around the jaws

● Chronic headaches or migraines

If you have any of these symptoms, see your dentist for advice.

What causes TMJ Syndrome?

As I said initially, no one fully understands TMJ. Both psychological and neurological factors may contribute to its causes. These, too, are poorly understood. The vast majority of TMJ sufferers are women. This further complicates the understanding of this problem, as purely physical causes should be evenly distributed among both sexes. Certain conditions, which I list below, often co-exist with TMJ and seem to explain the occurrence of the syndrome. Yet these same conditions may exist in other people who never have any symptoms of the problem!

A poor bite

The most common condition associated with TMJ Syndrome is a poor bite. A poor bite occurs when upper and lower teeth don't mesh correctly. This may be because the teeth are not aligned properly. That is, the teeth are

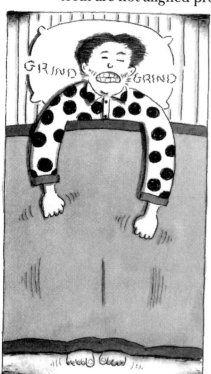

crowded and stick out in odd places and directions. Or, if teeth are missing and have not been replaced by bridges, implants, or dentures, the teeth will drift and lean, thereby interfering with a proper bite.

These poor bites force the jaws to close in a way that places a lot of strain and stress on the temporomandibular joints. Most people's joints are robust enough to handle this. Some people's joints, however, don't do so well under this kind of stress, and they develop problems and symptoms.

Grinding or clenching your teeth

Nervous habits, such as grinding or clenching teeth, especially during the night while sleeping, also stress these jaw joints and can result in TMJ problems.

Collapsed bites

A collapsed bite is the term used for a lower jaw which closes further than it is supposed to. Normally, the lower jaw closes until the upper and lower teeth meet. However, this normal stop is altered if a lot of teeth are missing or have tilted or drifted. As well, the lower jaw is allowed to close further than normal if full dentures have not been relined as the bone underneath them gradually disappears. This overclosure of the lower jaw stresses both TM joints.

Accidents

An accidental blow to the face may damage one or both TM joints and cause TMJ problems.

What causes the pain of TMJ Syndrome?

The stresses listed above either cause damage to the joints themselves or severely stress the muscles that control the joints. The pain comes from one of these sources.

If the joint has been damaged, it may become inflamed. Or, chronic stress on the joints may wear out some parts of them, causing pain. Or, arthritis may develop in the joint and lead to dramatic changes in its size and shape. This causes considerable pain, and greatly limits the functioning of the joint. Constant grinding and clenching of teeth can cause hyperactivity and stress in the muscles controlling the joints. The result is facial pain or migraines.

How is TMJ Syndrome treated?

The treatment for TMJ Syndrome varies from patient to patient. Treatment is very individualized because it depends on a careful evaluation of the underlying causes of the problem. There is no one treatment for everyone.

TMJ Syndrome can be treated in a number of ways. Relaxation training or psychological or psychiatric help may be the answer for patients grinding their teeth because of nervous stress. A plastic "nightguard" worn over the teeth at night provides smooth, gliding surfaces for the teeth and can eliminate the grinding because it leaves nothing for the teeth to grind on.

An **occlusal adjustment** may help when an improper bite is the cause. The dentist files down the offending teeth so that all teeth meet in harmony. The amount of filing is minimal and the procedure is painless. Sometimes several sessions are required over three to six months to correct the bite. Severely misaligned teeth may require orthodontic treatment to be placed in proper positions.

When missing, drifting, or tilting teeth are the cause of TMJ symptoms, they can be reconstructed with bridges, implants, or partial dentures to correct the problem.

Full mouth reconstruction may be the necessary solution if a collapsed bite is the problem. This involves replacing missing teeth, uprighting tilted ones, building up worn–down teeth or, if the patient has dentures, building up the old dentures or making new ones.

If the muscles controlling the TM joints are overtaxed, they may need to be treated first, before the bite is corrected. Heat treatments, exercises, and even steroid injections may be required. Oral anti-inflammatory medications and rest may also help.

A joint which is physically damaged may require surgery. This isn't as drastic as it sounds, thanks to new orthoscopic techniques. A small incision is made and a fiberoptic lens is inserted into the joint so that the dentist can get a closer look. Then a visually guided instrument can be used to correct the problem.

To sum up: The key to success with TMJ treatment is proper diagnosis of the cause. TMJ problems generally take many years to develop. They cannot be fixed overnight. Patience and understanding of the underlying reasons are essential. But don't give up. With proper treatment, most symptoms can be resolved.

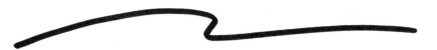

Geriatric dentistry

We're living longer — and we're keeping our teeth longer. The proportion of the population sixty-five years and older is expected to double between now and the year 2015, from ten percent to twenty percent of the populace. The age group seventy-five years and over is the single fastest growing segment of the population. And every ten years, the percentage of the elderly who have all or most of their own teeth rises dramatically. This is great news and a verification of what dentists have been saying for a long time: Teeth were meant to last a lifetime!

However, aging does present special concerns for dentists and patients alike.

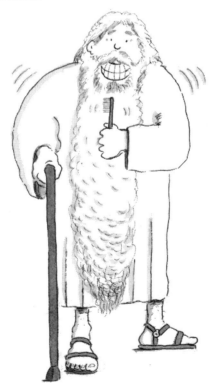

The most common problems of the aging mouth

The most common concerns of the silver-generation patient are periodontal disease, root cavities and soft tissue conditions.

Periodontal disease

Studies show that the incidence of periodontal (gum) disease neither increases nor decreases with age. This would suggest that periodontal disease is not a natural hazard of aging but, rather, a result of bacterial infection at any stage of life. However, there are some reasons that elderly people may be particularly susceptible to gum disease. The main weapon against gum disease is a meticulously clean mouth, and chronic conditions such as arthritis or nervous disorders may make it particularly difficult for older people to keep their mouths scrupulously clean. Aids such as floss handles and water irrigators may help maintain cleanliness. Electric toothbrushes may also help if motor skills are impaired.

More frequent cleaning visits to the dentist may be necessary to keep an eye on the situation, too. Anti-plaque rinses and anti-tartar toothpaste also may help.

Root caries

Older patients usually don't develop many new cavities. They are much more likely to suffer from recurrent decay around existing fillings. As well, since periodontal disease has had a longer time to develop around an older person's teeth, it may have caused gums to recede far enough to expose the roots of the teeth. These roots are not covered by strong enamel, so they are more susceptible to decay. The result is root cavities.

Root cavities are very common in older patients. They are more difficult to detect than regular cavities. This means that older patients require particularly thorough examinations when they come for a checkup. As well, root caries are more difficult to restore than regular cavities. Access in-between roots is limited. The walls of the roots containing the nerve canals of the teeth tend to be thin. This means that these nerves are often exposed as a result of even the shallowest root cavities. Frequent checkups are required to spot these cavities early, before they get too deep. If a nerve has been exposed, a root canal is necessary.

Fluoridation is important in controlling root caries. Drinking fluoridated water is crucial. The fluorides from the water are released around the gum of each tooth as well as in saliva. This means they are right in the area where they are needed most. Once absorbed onto the surface of the root, they greatly increase its resistance to decay. Topical fluoride treatments in the office, as well as home rinses, are of great benefit, too.

Soft tissues

Aging affects the soft tissues of the mouth. Mucous membranes tend to become frail and dry. Elderly people are particularly susceptible to mouth infections, too. Candida (a yeast infection) and mouth ulcers are very common. Antibiotics, widely used by elderly people for various other ailments, foster the growth of mouth infections such as these by killing off harmless bacteria and allowing more room for yeasts and the like to multiply.

The incidence of oral cancers also increases with age. Men are twice as susceptible as women are to contract mouth cancer, partly because they smoke more. Chronic irritation to the gums from ill-fitting dentures may also lead to the formation of mouth tumors.

Chronic conditions such as these can usually be prevented through good denture maintenance by patient and dentist. Regular checkups, relines, and refittings of faulty dentures are essential.

The best weapon against all these diseases is early detection. Frequent, regular dental checkups are a must — even when no natural teeth are present.

Dry Mouth (xerostomia)

Another common condition in the aging patient is **xerostomia** or **dry mouth.** There are many causes of this condition. Hundreds of medications cause mouth dryness as a side effect. Some of the most common of these are sedatives and medications used to control hypertension and Parkinson's disease.

Generalized conditions such as internal bleeding, vomiting, or persistent diarrhea also may cause dryness of the mouth.

Diseases that directly affect the salivary glands can also cause a decrease in saliva production, which leads to xerostomia.

What are the symptoms of dry mouth?
The most common symptoms of dry mouth are a sore mouth and a burning tongue. Dry mouth causes a rapid increase in the incidence of cavities. I have several patients in my practice for whom I can't provide fillings fast enough. Even if I see them every two months for a checkup, I still discover several new teeth decaying at each visit. If these unfortunate people lose teeth, they find wearing dentures almost impossible because of the lack of saliva in their mouths. The rubbing and irritation is extreme.

How is dry mouth treated?
Lubricants such as Orajel can help alleviate the symptoms, but there is no real cure for dry mouth. Synthetic saliva such as Xerolube is particularly good because it contains fluoride. Sugarless candy or gum helps, too. Regular mouth rinses should be avoided because they contain alcohol which further dries out the mouth.

The elderly patient with full dentures
The bony ridges of the jaws are maintained by the presence of teeth. These ridges resorb (dissolve and assimilate) over time once teeth are gone. This makes it difficult to wear full dentures, especially in the lower jaw. In some older patients, the bone resorption is so advanced that certain internal nerves in the lower jaw are no longer encased in bone but, instead, are covered with gum tissue only. The pressure from dentures leaning on these exposed nerves can cause excruciating pain.

Soreness under dentures develops rapidly since elderly people's tissues tend to be thin and frail. It is often advisable to make "soft-bottom" dentures for these people. The underside of soft-bottom dentures is made of a soft, elastic-rubber compound that provides great comfort.

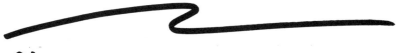

Glossary

Abscess
A sack-like accumulation of pus, debris, and bacteria found around a damaged or injured tooth.

Amalgam, silver
A metal alloy, containing silver, mercury, and small quantities of other metals, used for filling dental cavities. Commonly called a silver filling.

Analgesics
Medications designed to reduce pain. Popularly known as pain-killers.

Anesthetic
A type of medication designed to temporarily numb (freeze) a particular area of the body.

Ankylosis
A dental condition in which the tooth fuses directly to the jaw-bone, without the normal, cushioning, soft tissues (gum liga-ments) in-between. Most commonly occurs after an accidental blow.

Antibiotics
A type of medication designed to kill bacterial infections in the body. In dentistry, used mainly to resolve tooth abscesses or gum infections.

Assignment
Refers to assigning insurance benefits to the dentist. The insurance company pays the dentist directly for any treatment performed.

Bleaching
A method of whitening teeth by using special solutions.

Bonding
A method of attaching dental restorations to teeth. Bonding can be used to attach white fillings, veneers, crowns, bridges or orthodontic braces.

Braces
Small brackets made of metal, plastic, or porcelain, and attached to teeth by bonding or metal bands for the purpose of straightening or aligning teeth.

Bridge
A permanent prosthetic (artificial) device made to replace one or more missing teeth. Attaches to existing teeth on either side of the space.

Bruxism
A condition in which patients grind their teeth, usually at night or at times of stress. Results in the wearing down of the teeth.

Calculus
Hard, calcified matter that collects on teeth if they are not cleaned properly. Consists of calcified (hardened) plaque or debris, bacteria, and protein molecules from saliva. Commonly known as **tartar** or stone.

Cap
Common name for a crown.

Caries
Dental term for a cavity.

Cavity
A defect (hole) in a tooth caused by bacterial acids in plaque.

Cementum
A substance covering the root portion of the tooth. In a healthy tooth, cementum is completely embedded in the jawbone and covered by gum.

Cephalometric X-ray
A special profile X-ray of the entire head showing the relationship between the jaws and the rest of the skull. Important during diagnosis prior to orthodontic treatment.

Collapsed bite
A condition in which the lower jaw closes further than is normal. Caused by missing, leaning, or poorly-positioned teeth.

Cross-bite
A situation where one or more of the lower teeth overlap the upper ones.

Crown
A dental restoration that completely covers, strengthens, and protects the entire tooth.

Dentin
A hard, bonelike, yellow substance that makes up the bulk of the tooth. In the crown part it is covered by enamel, and in the root portion; by cementum.

Denture
A removable prosthetic (artificial) device designed to replace some or all missing teeth in the upper or lower jaw.

Disclosing tablets
Tablets containing vegetable dye, used to reveal areas of the teeth where brushing needs improvement.

Drill
See handpiece.

Dry sockets
A painful condition which sometimes occurs after a tooth extraction. Normal healing is halted because the blood clot has been lost at the site of the tooth extraction. Requires prompt dental attention.

Enamel
A hard white substance covering the crown portion of a tooth. Enamel is the hardest substance in the body.

Endondontics/Endodontist
A dental specialty/specialist dealing with root canal treatment.

Erupt/Eruption
Breaking of a new tooth through the gum and the subsequent growth of the tooth into proper position in the jaw.

Filling
A restoration material placed in a tooth cavity to repair it and return the tooth to its original size, form, and function.

Fluoride
A naturally-occurring chemical element which, when incorporated into tooth tissues, makes them more resistant to cavity formation.

Freeze
See anesthetic.

Gingiva
The soft tissue surrounding the teeth commonly known as the gum.

Gingivitis
An inflammation of the gums. Usually the first stage of periodontal disease.

Handpiece
Dental term referring to a drill. A handpiece shapes and cleans teeth to prepare them for restorations.

Headgear
An orthodontic appliance made of thick wire connected to the upper back teeth, and extending to an elastic connected to a neck strap or a small skullcap. It is intended to pull the upper jaw and teeth backwards to correct a skeletal discrepancy between the upper and lower jaws.

Hygienist
A dental professional who looks after the health of the teeth and gums. The dental hygienist cleans the teeth, and removes plaque and calculus.

Impacted Tooth/Impaction
A condition in which teeth are not positioned properly in the jawbone during their formation. As a result, they cannot properly erupt into the mouth.

Implant
Foreign material, usually metal, surgically embedded in the jawbone to act as a foundation for the replacement of missing teeth.

Impression
An indent of the teeth made by using a special, rubber-like material. From this indent, plaster models of teeth can be cast to make prostheses (artificial teeth) or restorations (tooth repairs).

Infection
An invasion and penetration of body tissues by micro-organisms such as bacteria or viruses.

Inflammation
An aggravated state of body tissues caused by irritation or physical stress.

Inlays
A type of tooth filling prepared in a laboratory, usually made of gold or porcelain.

Laughing gas
Nitrous oxide gas used to calm a nervous patient during a dental treatment visit. Laughing gas is inhaled by the patient as a relaxant during the appointment. It quickly wears off afterward.

Leaky fillings
Old fillings that have lost their integrity and no longer provide a tight seal to the tooth. Bacteria collects between the filling and the tooth, causing further decay and destruction of the tooth.

Maxillo-facial surgeon
See oral surgeon.

Mercury
Quicksilver, a toxic chemical element. Used as a component of silver amalgam fillings. Recent evidence questions the advisability of its use in dental fillings.

Nightguard
A removable, clear plastic appliance worn over all the upper or lower teeth to prevent bruxism (grinding of teeth).

Onlays
A laboratory-fabricated tooth restoration that fills and restores a defect in the tooth. It extends over the edges of the defect to hold the remaining parts of the tooth together, thereby strengthening the tooth. Usually made of gold or porcelain.

Open contact
A condition in which two neighboring teeth fail to touch each other. Food and other matter collect in such an opening, damaging the teeth and surrounding gums.

Open bite
A condition in which upper and lower front teeth do not meet.

Oral surgeon
A dental specialist concerned with correcting jawbone deformities resulting from birth defects or accidents, and with difficult tooth extractions. Also called a maxillo-facial surgeon.

Orthodontics/Orthodontist
The dental specialty/specialist concerned with straightening and alignment of teeth.

Overbite
A vertical overlap of front teeth.

Pedodontics/Pedodontist
Children's dentistry/dentist.

Periodontal disease
Gum disease.

Periodontics/Periodontist
The dental specialty/specialist concerned with the treatment of gum disease and gum problems.

Plaque
A whitish film that accumulates on teeth which are not brushed regularly. Consists of bacteria, food remnants, debris, and protein molecules in saliva.

Pocket
A groove between the tooth and the surrounding gum which has deepened to more than the normal, healthy three millimetres.

Prosthesis
An artificial appliance such as a bridge, denture, or implant, used to replace missing teeth.

Prosthodontics/Prosthodontist
A dental specialty/specialist dealing with prosthetic (artificial) tooth replacement.

Proxibrush
A small brush used to clean in-between teeth and around crowns and bridges. Also called an interproximal brush.

Recontouring
Selective filing of parts of teeth to improve their cosmetic appearance.

Relines
A method of refitting dentures so that the underside of the dentures closely adapts once again to the tissues of the jaw on which it rests.

Resin
Another name for a white or tooth-colored filling material.

Retainer
An orthodontic appliance worn for several months after orthodontic treatment is complete. Its function is to hold the teeth in their new positions and to prevent them from relapsing.

Rheumatic fever
A condition that sometimes follows a bout of scarlet fever. Patients with this condition must be treated with antibiotics before each dental treatment.

Root caries
Cavities that develop on the roots of teeth. They usually occur in older patients, or in patients whose gums have receded from periodontal disease, which exposes the roots.

Root canal
A dental treatment involving the removal of diseased soft tissues from inside the tooth.

Root planing
Cleaning of root surfaces exposed by periodontal disease. Performed to get rid of calculus and to smooth irregularities.

S. mutans
Streptococci mutans, a particular species of bacteria that feeds on sugars and excretes acid strong enough to dissolve tooth enamel. These are the bacteria responsible for tooth decay.

Scaling
A process of removing hard calculus (tartar) from the surfaces of teeth.

Serial extractions
A method of timed and selective extraction of baby teeth to prevent anticipated crowding of permanent teeth. When timed well, serial extractions reduce the need for subsequent orthodontic treatment.

Shedding
Natural loss of baby teeth as permanent teeth begin to erupt.

Skeletal problems
Disharmony between the size and the rate of growth of upper and lower jaws. This leads to an improper bite between upper and lower teeth and necessitates orthodontic treatment.

Soft tissues
Any non-bony parts of the body, such as blood vessels, nerves, muscles, gums.

Space maintainer
A device designed to hold the space of a prematurely lost baby tooth until the permanent tooth erupts.

Space regaining appliance
A device used to push drifted teeth back to their normal position in order to allow space for a new permanent tooth space to erupt.

Tartar
Common name for calculus.

TMJ
Temporomandibular joint. One of two joints located just in front of each ear. These joints hinge the lower jaw to the upper one.

TMJ Syndrome
A complex and painful condition involving the temporomandibular joints and surrounding muscles.

Veneer
Thin facing bonded to the visible part of the tooth to improve its cosmetic appearance.

White filling
A plastic-type filling material that matches the color of the tooth.

Wisdom teeth
The four back molar teeth, one in each corner of the upper and lower jaw. The wisdom teeth are normally the last teeth to erupt. They usually appear in the mouth between the ages of sixteen and twenty-one years.

Xerostomia
A condition of dry mouth. The production of saliva is stopped or reduced due to primary gland disease or as a side effect of some medications.

Index